FROM ANECDOTE
TO ANTIDOTE

FROM ANECDOTE TO ANTIDOTE

Medical Musings and Practical Prescriptions from a Humanitarian Healer

Richard Klein, M.D.

SelectBooks, Inc.
New York

First Edition

ISBN 978-1-59079-151-6

Library of Congress Cataloging-in-Publication Data

Klein, Richard S. , 1938–

From anecdote to antidote : medical musings and practical prescriptions from a humanitarian healer / Richard S. Klein. -- 1st ed.

p. cm.

ISBN 978-1-59079-151-6 (pbk. : alk. paper)

1. Medicine--Anecdotes. 2. Physicians--Anecdotes. 3. Physician and patient--Anecdotes. I. Title.

R705.K66 2008

610--dc22

2008017127

Manufactured in the United States of America

10 9 8 7 6 5 4 3 2 1

This book is dedicated to the memory of Brian Klein and the sadness of his passing; and to my wife, Caryn—to our family and the brightness of our lives.

ACKNOWLEDGMENTS

I would like to thank Dee DelBello for the encouragement to write this book. Thanks also to Marci Smith, Robert Rozycki, and most especially to Derek Rydall, without whose help this task would never have succeeded.

CONTENTS

INTRODUCTION

What a Doctor Knows (Could Fill Life's Waiting Room)

AT A CERTAIN POINT IN ONE'S LIFE one can develop a crystalline knowledge. Stevie Nicks of Fleetwood Mac likened this clarity, this crystalline clarity, to the cleanness of water. It's an ability to clearly know and understand life. To learn from its ups and downs. To feel through the experiences of others. If I were to give this development a diagnosis, I would most likely call it, "Knowledgitis."

Best part is, I think I have it! (Okay, okay … it's a self-diagnosis, but it works for me.) After years and years as a successful physician, I believe some of what I've learned should be passed on to make the learning curve for the rest of us so much easier. I believe that patients and their doctors can benefit from what I've observed personally, overheard second-hand, or just plain absorbed in my thirty-plus years in the medical profession.

Gauging from my early beginnings, one would never have thought I would be where I am today. I was born and raised in the tenements of the Lower East Side of New York City. I chose playing hooky to schooling. So I dropped out and joined the U.S. Navy, then the U.S. Marine Corps. By following the flow of the river of life, I wound up a medical student in Italy. There, I ultimately found myself as I fell in love with the country and embraced its culture.

Since then I've volunteered as a physician in two of the Arab-Israeli wars, achieved knighthood, and made an unfortunately unsuccessful run for the U.S. Congress seat for New York's 19th Congressional District. I've met a pope on two occasions, as well as a U.S. president. I've dined with prime ministers, presidents, and generals of foreign countries.

Not bad for a city kid.

My thirty-some-odd years of practicing medicine have taught me about the preciousness of life and how tenuous it is. Life is so, so short to spend our days in the kind of worries and pursuits that, in the face of death, matter very little. Of the many deathly ill patients that I've admitted to the hospital, never did one say, "Doctor, I didn't go to work enough. Doctor, I didn't rearrange my sock drawer enough. Doctor, I didn't pay my bills early enough. Doctor, I didn't watch enough TV." It was always, "Doctor, I didn't take time to smell the roses."

Rabbi David Greenberg of Temple Shaaray Tefila, in Bedford, NY, said it so eloquently this past Yom Kippur. In his Day of Atonement sermon, he reminded all of a bumper sticker he once saw which read, "Don't postpone joy." If I had room enough, I would print up the following bumper sticker (or maybe it should be a billboard in Times Square): "Don't take life for granted. Don't take health for granted. Don't take for granted that you can recapture in the future the goodness and the beauty that is available to you today and, hopefully, tomorrow."

It's a shame that all too often it takes a tragedy or encounter with death to make us want to do something about life. How many families have I heard express regret after a loved one's passing that they never told them they loved them or, if they had, that they hadn't said it enough?

I suppose much of my rationale for putting these thoughts down on paper is to save my readers some of those regrets. Not every anecdote on the following pages is about doom and gloom—there are plenty of hearts and flowers along the way—but every one is a potential reflection upon life versus death.

I agree with the rabbi when he states, "When we look back upon our lives, we will regret the things that we didn't do more than the ill conceived things that we did do. We will recognize that most of our disappointments in life were the result not of efforts gone wrong, but of efforts that were never made." It's upsetting that people don't work to fulfill their dreams, that they procrastinate about their health or their desired vocations, that they hesitate to express emotions or reach out to distant family, friends, or lovers. Some blame others or circumstances for their failures; some just drop out.

The other day, a local high school class graduated. The valedictorian was a girl from Bangladesh. Her family escaped poverty and hunger, coming to their relatives' house here in New York just four years ago. I thought of how hard that young girl had to work, coming from such a disadvantaged country, to become the top of her class. She was given the same opportunities as all of her classmates, just as all of us in this country are given the same opportunity. Therefore, all of us potentially have the same chance of being successful. And yet many of us fall into the same old ruts, scrambling for purchase high atop the rung of that ladder to success and ignoring the bigger opportunities for personal growth along the way.

In *From Anecdote to Antidote* I try to share my favorite stories from thirty years in the medical profession. I thought I could just arrange them willy-nilly, allowing my pearls of wisdom to string you along from beginning to end, but as I moved forward through the initial draft I found that most of the stories fell into one of three categories, with a special bonus wrap-up section at the end:

PART 1: *People*—covering not only some of the more fascinating people I've met my through my career, famous and not, but delving into the humanity of us all, doctors included, with warts and imperfections fully exposed

PART 2: *Places*—concerning the places I have been on my journey though life and learning; places not just physical, but also existential; places where not all of us have been, but where, perhaps, all of us could go

PART 3: *Things*—a compendium of practical knowledge designed to help you both maintain health and navigate the road of life we all travel, as well as the detours that some of us must sometimes take

Throughout, I do my best to communicate the lessons I've learned along the way from all of these people, places, and things. As you read along, I think you'll find the table of contents useful as the stories tend to lend themselves to the general themes I've mapped out for you. But by the same token there is a universality, I feel, to all of the stories.

Yes, I've grouped them into themes and sub-themes, afflictions and aspirations, but when you're done with the book I hope you'll agree with me that they all fall under that universal condition we call life.

For what is a doctor if not a saver—a reminder—of human life?

PART 1

PEOPLE

Introduction

*"It is healthy to be reminded that the strongest might weaken
and the wisest might err."*

—MOHANDAS K. (MAHATMA) GANDHI

ONE OF MY MAIN GOALS WITH this book is to ease the intimidation I see in my patients' eyes as I consult with them for the first time. Not because I don't enjoy being put on a pedestal (I do), but because of how it influences their behavior while we discuss such important things as their medical history, weight, allergies, past medical procedures, et cetera. I can't tell you how many second opinions I've given, often in complete reversal of a previous doctor's diagnosis, that could have been easily avoided if the patients had simply been more honest and less intimidated by their doctor during their initial consultation.

I can understand the sense of intimidation. Sometimes people feel uncomfortable or insecure around someone who may have had a more extensive education than they have. And, as in any human situation, there is the issue of "power." Think about it: you're entrusting your health and well-being into the hands of someone outside your family, someone you don't know, someone who (in most cases) went to school for an additional eight years after college and regularly cut into corpses as practice for tending to your healthcare needs. On top of which, you're sitting there in his office, on his turf, in a paper dress with your rear end hanging out.

Of course, I could tell you the many ways in which doctors are people. We take out our own trash, do our own shopping, mop our own floors, even stand in front of the over-the-counter drug aisle, just as perplexed as you are, when we have a runny nose or stomach ache.

We forge relationships with patients, develop individual likes and dislikes, and can often both sympathize and empathize with those in our care. We fall in and out of love, go through mid-life crises, keep hobbies, and pursue interests—like, say, writing a book—and we (hopefully) learn something from each interaction and experience. But as my creative writing teacher once told me (or should I say, told me many, many dozens of times), "it's better to show than tell."

So here's where I start. By recounting the people I've met over the course of my career on the following pages, and recounting the things I've learned from them, I will *show* you the many ways in which doctors, mainly myself, are more human than one might expect and far more fallible than people give us credit for. It is not my hope to throw egg on my face or the faces of my colleagues, but instead to inspire you to be more confident, brave, and forthcoming the next time you're sitting across from your own doctor and telling him about your various aches and ills.

I could tell you to picture him in his underwear, but I know that's pretty hard to do when you're sitting there in yours. So instead I'll show you, time and again, that doctors are human too.

The Art of Medicine

As THEY WERE LEAVING THE OFFICE, a patient of mine, Mr. Davis, proudly pointed to his wife Naomi and announced to the office staff that they were celebrating their 60th wedding anniversary that day. A round of applause went up for the beaming couple.

I asked, "Do you have any words of wisdom as to your marriage's success?"

"Well," he replied, "you have to hear a little less than you really do, and see less than there really is."

These words should not only be the mantra of all newlyweds, but of friends in general.

Conversely, it takes years of practice to realize that it's more important to listen to what a patient is saying than it is to quickly reel off what might be wrong. There is a fine line between hearing and listening. Some people watch the other person's lips move and call it "hearing." Others wait until the other person stops speaking so they can interject and call that "listening." But just as there's a gulf of difference between the individual examples I've offered, there's an ocean between hearing and actually listening to what the speaker is trying to convey. Obviously, listening transcends medicine and is one of the most important tools we have in communicating with our fellow human beings.

Looking back, this might be my greatest lesson of all and, in the early years, my biggest source of mistakes.

During my introduction to Physical Diagnosis in my second year of medical school in Rome, I met my professor, Dr. Antonio Carrozza. Professor Carrozza was as round and comforting as his name (which means "carriage" in Italian), always exuding a fatherly warmth and jovial nature, as well as a perpetual smile. He taught the men and women sitting in his class that ninety-eight percent of a patient's diagnosis would come from just sitting there and listening. And, of course, asking the right questions. Once, when asked what test or instrument he would need to help his patients if he were to set up an office in a small, isolated village, Professor Carrozza answered, "a chair."

Sadly, this basic yet highly effective approach is eclipsed in modern medicine and quite a bit of modern doctoring by a too-strong faith in cold machines performing CAT scans, MRIs, and blood tests. The *art* of medicine still lays in listening and observing your patient. Despite the sound of it, this is not always an easy task. There are times when a patient will ramble on and on about every possible symptom imaginable. "Well, doc, I have this cough. It's kind of a dry hack, and it gets so bad that I get stomach pains from coughing so hard and it makes me see stars. That makes me rub my eyes and shake my head to clear my vision, but then I get dizzy, so I go lie down and, before I know it, I'm asleep. Then I usually wake up an hour later and I'm all disoriented for a few minutes. So I make a pot of coffee but, when I drink it, I burn my tongue. And did I tell you that my right foot hurts?" By the time he's done, the patient is sure he's got lung cancer, glaucoma, narcolepsy, and Alzheimer's disease. Before the eyes start to glaze over, a well-trained physician will refocus the discussion. And the listening should not stop. Though a patient with every symptom under the sun is either a hypochondriac or one sick cookie, each one still requires a diagnosis at the end of his or her rambling.

Unfortunately, there are some patients who have difficulty explaining their symptoms or themselves. Rather than trying a different way to make themselves understood, they raise their voices, thinking you just cannot hear them clearly. I remember spending Thanksgiving in a small Florida town some years ago. We stopped at a gas station, and while refueling I noticed a restaurant that was across the street. The name was "Calypso" and I couldn't figure out by its name alone if it would be appropriate for traditional Thanksgiving fare. I asked the attendant what kind of restaurant it was and he said it was a "good restaurant."

Seeing that this was not quite the type of answer I was seeking, I asked again. This time the attendant raised his voice and said "I said it was a good restaurant and they serve very good food." You could see the exasperation of this young man, forced to deal with an out-of-towner—or a simpleton ... after all, how many different types of restaurants are there beyond good ones and bad ones?—who was also hard of hearing.

The problem was obviously one of communication. When faced with such a situation, a good physician should be calming and expert in drawing out the necessary information.

One of my dearest friends, Don, is a short, robust, sedentary older man who has been plagued with knee pains for the past few years. He eventually saw an orthopedist and a rheumatologist, and was found to have severe arthritis of both knees. What followed was a series of painful injections, intense physical therapy and, subsequently, arthroscopic surgery. Nothing seemed to alleviate the pain, and he ended up in such discomfort that his orthopedic specialists eventually recommended surgical knee replacement.

One day while we were having lunch together, he told me that despite this latest diagnosis, he never really got truly severe pains in his knees. After walking a few blocks, however, he said they ached. This wasn't the scenario for bilateral knee replacements, so I finally listened and at last started to hear what my friend was really telling me. It seemed that Don's real problem was weakness in his thighs, most probably from lower back disc disease. After our luncheon I arranged for Don to have an MRI of his lumbar spine. Sure enough, test results showed that he had significant disc disease with compression of his spinal cord. This, rather than faulty knees, was the cause of his disability.

Yes, there was arthritis of his knees but that wasn't what was *really* bothering him. He nearly got sold two new knees when all he needed was physical therapy to strengthen his back.

There is an art to get people to listen, whether it's in giving an order to a waiter or telling your mechanic about that "whirr" in the engine. One place you should always feel like you're being heard is your doctor's office. Sometimes, to be heard, there are specific methods to use when talking to a doctor or anyone in a similar position—teacher, clergyman, spouse, or (heaven forbid) a lawyer. One method to employ, perhaps the best, is to do some "homework." A little inquisitive reading about your symptoms and presumed situation can go a long way toward leveling the playing field, as well as show your doctor that you're ready to be an active player in your own upkeep—a situation that is far from universal. Do some research, perhaps draw up a list of questions to ask your doctor in advance.

Beyond that, don't be intimidated by the person or the scenario. Look your doctor in the eye when speaking with him, and don't be afraid to show concern; let him know you're an active partner in this project. And, most important, do not let your questions go unanswered. If an issue hasn't been resolved to the point of you truly feeling heard and understanding the response, press the matter. If that doesn't get results , or worse, if it obviously irritates a doctor, it may be time for a new doctor. Or at least a second opinion.

• • •

Equally important as both listening and being heard is keeping one's eyes opened to actually observe the situation. Or the willingness to do so.

When I was a medical student and intern, congestive heart failure was a gravely serious condition and very nearly a guaranteed death sentence. Congestive heart failure is characterized by the welling-up of fluid in the lungs and extremities, which then interferes with breathing, blood flow, and the very ability of the heart to beat. Because it is a systemic condition, affecting nearly the entire body, treating it posed a particular difficulty. Short of cutting a patient into pieces and wringing him out like a washcloth, there were few effective treatments for such an affliction. The generally accepted remedy was to place tourniquets on three of the four extremities and then rotate them every fifteen minutes. Imagine treating people with rotating tourniquets in a modern emergency room!

Or imagine, if you will, treating them with some of the most toxic elements occurring in nature. As horrifying as it may sound to some today, heavy metals were used in the pre-antibiotic and pre-steroidal era to treat a number of conditions. Some of these metals, such as arsenic, induced high fevers that killed susceptible organisms (syphilis, for one). Around the time we were treating congestive heart failure with tourniquets, my New York Medical College professor, Dr. George Vogel, and his colleagues noticed that the patients being treated for certain diseases with the heavy metal mercury started urinating a lot.

This observation that mercury induced urination when given to patients with congestive heart failure, thus relieving their breathing by causing diuresis (doctor-speak for increased urine flow), led to the production of one of the first manufactured diuretics: Mercuhydrin. This was quickly followed by many other diuretic drugs. And, of course, we said goodbye to tourniquet therapy.

As we all know (I would hope), the fields of medicine and health-care are continually evolving, just as the above anecdote illustrates.

Treatments that were previously considered cutting edge, such as lobotomy, Thalidomide and Vioxx, regularly fall by the wayside as the result of diligent observation and inquisitiveness, the true mothers of invention. Unfortunately, these two simple yet effective traits are often shouldered aside when physicians—with the best of intentions, mind you—are so sure of a diagnosis or preferred regimen of treatment that they fail to do the "busy work" that would allow them to see the forest for the trees. Or, in this case, the malady for the symptoms.

I recently reviewed a malpractice claim where a family physician wrongly treated his patient for a urinary tract infection. The patient had undergone a prostate biopsy one week before and now had fever. The physician noted that there were red blood cells in the patient's urine, which is very common after a prostate biopsy. He did not note, however, any white blood cells in that same specimen, which is a sign of infection. Nor did he confirm any infection by obtaining a urine culture. The prescribed oral antibiotics did help, but two weeks later the fever came back. Again, without checking the urine, another series of antibiotics was ordered, and then a third. The patient ultimately suffered a massive stroke after an infected piece of fibrotic tissue broke loose from his heart and clogged a major brain artery.

The patient originally was suffering from an infected heart valve, which became infected at the time of the prostate biopsy. The prescribed oral antibiotics were no match for this serious infection. The physician also never got his head out of the sand. He thought the patient had a urinary tract infection, but never observed proof of this.

As another example, last year my wife's grandmother Ruth developed fevers and swelling around her recently replaced artificial knee following a fall. Her local small town orthopedist guessed, correctly, that she suffered with a knee infection and immediately started her on intravenous antibiotics. The treatment lasted six weeks, which was appropriate. What was not appropriate was the fact that the doctor never did any culturing; he believed the infecting organism was due to a particular bacteria and that's what he treated her for. When her fevers returned after the six weeks of treatment, his treatment was to repeat the same antibiotic again.

Trying to gently encourage an elderly patient to get another opinion is extremely difficult, if not impossible. Ruth lived in this small community for years and was loyal to her physicians. As far as she was concerned, they could do no wrong. (If only she had read the previous anecdote!) The family knew things were amiss, but nobody could convince grandmother. Ruth did agree to our suggestion that she see an infectious disease consultant, but the first consultant called by the orthopedist wouldn't see her because the convalescent home Ruth was being treated in was too far away. The second I.D. doctor should have staid away. Much to my chagrin, she continued the same therapeutic course. After four months of the same see-saw regimen with no results, Ruth finally gave in. She was transferred to an orthopedic hospital where all antibiotics were stopped for two weeks. Cultures were then obtained which revealed the real culprit, which was quite different than that assumed by her community physician. The infection was finally eradicated and Ruth can walk and dance once more. Stubborn loyalty to a physician, who was stubborn himself for not getting his head out of the sand, led to an unnecessary four-months of suffering.

• • •

Since we've already established the importance of being heard by your doctor, I also want to emphasize how important it is to be proactive in the maintenance of your own health to add strength to your voice. We're just as responsible as our physicians, and must know as much as we can and must stay informed about issues that relate to our health. You and only you are the best barometer of the goings on in your own body, you know best when you feel normal and when you don't. But a doctor is almost always the best source of help if and when something does go wrong. And though our skills are many (if I do say so myself), we are not mind readers and can't just look at you and tell what you're thinking, what's bothering you, and what exactly is wrong. So you should never be afraid to ask your doctor a so-called "stupid" question, make a "dumb" suggestion, or offer an observation that seems so "obvious." Do not hesitate to share any information you've discovered, hunches you may have, or "scuttle-butt" you've heard about relevant health issues with your doctor.

As difficult as it is to suffer with a malady, or even the fear of one, it is more difficult to suffer in fear of the unknown. It is an unfortunate fact of life that disease happens. Fortunately, most diseases are curable if found early. If you take a positive approach to disease and are open with your doctor, you have a much higher chance of being one of the fortunate. You may or may not open the door—and your doctor's eyes—to a new avenue of treatment, but you'll demonstrate your own level of commitment to your own health (something doctors appreciate and welcome), and go a long way to livening up those dry, clinical conversations.

The Arnold Palmer Syndrome:
"The More I Play,
The Luckier I Become" [1]

HOW AM I DOING SO FAR? Considering that my stated purpose is to convince you, the reader, of a doctor's basic humanity, I'd like to think I'm at least doing well enough. We've taken the doctor off of his artificial pedestal and initiated a level conversation between doctor and patient, two sentient , fragile, fallible human beings. What could be more human than that?

How about a plainly stated belief in luck? Whether you call it "coincidence," "kismet," a "happy accident," or what have you, it has been such a recurring matter in my life and career that I cannot discount it, regardless of how supernaturally freaky it may sound.

Years ago, the Armenian Bishop of Jerusalem, Giuregh Kapikian, came to my office in Yorktown to surprise me with a visit. I had become quite friendly with him during my many visits to Jerusalem and through my many efforts to help that city's Armenian community after Israel's reunification of the Holy City in 1967. Perhaps one of the most memorable instances from my work with the Armenians was when I was able to use my friendship with Deputy Mayor Lotte Salzberger and Mayor Teddy Kollek to allow the Armenians to march during the anniversary of the Great Calamity, their genocide at the hands of the Ottoman Turks during World War I. For years the Israeli government would not allow the Armenians a sanctioned public commemoration in deference to Turkey. At that time, Turkey was the only Muslim country maintaining diplomatic ties with Israel.

I hadn't seen the bishop in a year. He had always been a robust, smiling, energetic dynamo of a man, but when he walked in he looked to be anything but. He was pale, gaunt, and had about him an aroma of *melena*, a foul, pervasive, nostril-lingering indicator of digested blood (*melena*, from the Greek "black," denotes dark tar-like

---

[1] When congratulated on a particularly great shot, the great golfer simply claimed it was luck and then gave this marvelous quote.

stool formed from the enzymatic breakdown of blood from the upper gastrointestinal system).

During my first year at the University of Rome studying physical diagnosis, one of the first tools taught to us in examining a patient was our sense of smell. We smelled the mouth and body of diabetics, patients in kidney or liver failure, and patients with gastrointestinal bleeds. Because even the patients are familiar with their own different body smells, honing that sense of smell adds another dimension in solving the puzzle and aids our ears when they alone can't "hear" what's wrong with an undiagnosed patient. (Speaking of humanity, it is vital that a doctor incorporate all of the senses in evaluating a patient. As a patient walks by, one can see if they are limping or if their body shape has changed; a change in the scent of one's natural body odor or breath can indicate any number of conditions. And of course we're always poking and prodding our patients and listening to their lungs and heartbeats. I can only hope that it does not become conventional practice to start tasting blood and urine samples in an effort to determine intoxication or blood sugar levels.)

I asked Bishop Kapikian if I could do a blood count and, upon finding a severe anemia, he consented to a rectal test. Not the kind of greeting you would expect from a long lost friend. The diagnosis was sobering to the both of us: colon cancer. Obviously I was terribly worried for my friend. After having not seen him for so long, the wonderful surprise of his unannounced visit was far outweighed by the gravity of this just-discovered situation. But Bishop Kapikian, ever the man of faith, simply said, "I am in God's hands."

As it turned out, his colon cancer was found in time and he lived for years and years after that lucky surprise visit, often kidding about how my saving his life gave him renewed zeal in preaching his religion. For years, the bishop and his New York family and I teased and kidded each other about the fact that a Jewish doctor inspired proselytizing by the Orthodox Church.

• • •

Paying attention to your body with all your senses can give you vital clues to your overall health, motivate you to pay a visit to your family physician, and make the difference between longevity and disease. Your body is an amazing vehicle; like the instrument panel in your car, it is constantly giving you readouts of your health and well-being, telling you when you need to slow down, fill up, change your oil, get your engine tuned, or get a complete overhaul. If you pay attention to what your body is telling you and don't take any strange sounds or funny smells for granted, you will recognize most problems before they cause you to overheat, stall in traffic, or run off the road into a ditch!

And a little luck never hurts, either. In Bishop Kapikian's case, we were both lucky, he because he managed to have a life-threatening condition caught before it was too late, and me because I was able to help save the life of a dear friend. That experience also taught us a lesson: be on the lookout for advice wherever and whenever you can find it. You never know when sound medical counsel is right around the corner. Or, for that matter, at the bottom of your ladder.

When I recently had my home stereo system upgraded, the manager of the local electronics store, a nice guy named Mark, was running all sorts of wires all over the house to connect all of the far flung speakers. When he climbed up a ladder, I noticed an ugly growth on his leg and asked Mark how long he had it.

"About eleven or twelve months," he replied. "And it seems to be getting bigger." Well, that was a mean-looking lesion that had the menacing features of a melanoma, the most dreaded of skin cancers. Mark lived in Brooklyn but asked if I could recommend a local surgeon, for I insisted that the lesion be biopsied. It took him a month or so to call the surgeon, but after he did the biopsy proved positive for melanoma. Shortly thereafter Mark was undergoing MRIs and CT scans to see if the cancer had spread.

Unfortunately, his liver and spleen were studded with melanoma. The expert at Memorial Sloan Kettering couldn't help him, so we arranged for a trip to the National Institutes of Health in Maryland. There, a Dr. Rosenberg was doing some experimental therapy. Though considered too toxic for older patients, Mark was considered a viable candidate for the trial because he was still shy of his thirtieth birthday. In this case, time really was on Mark's side. His lesions melted away under Dr. Rosenberg's experimental protocol, which is almost unheard of for conventional chemotherapy of metastatic, terminal melanoma.

With a new lease on life Mark quit the stereo business, got married, and is moving to Colorado. He decided to change careers and is enrolling in pharmacy school, all because I needed help with the master power controls to my stereo.

• • •

Fifteen years ago, my staff and I were just getting ready to close the office and go home when Ray Carino appeared at the front door. Ray was pale, drenched in perspiration and obviously in pain. My nurse Jackie helped me to get him into an examining room, and as I helped undress Ray and took his vitals I told Jackie to get an EKG. I informed the secretary that no matter what, Ray was going to need to be admitted to the hospital and asked her to call for an ambulance.

After the few minutes it took to hook him up and start running the tracing, we could see evidence of a massive heart attack. Then, suddenly, his heart went into the dreaded ventricular fibrillation, a condition where the heart muscle goes into spasm rather than continuing to pump blood through the circulatory system. I had been in practice twenty years and never, ever had a patient go into ventricular fibrillation in my office. I therefore never needed or purchased a defibrillator, a device that delivers electric shocks to break the electrical "short circuit" causing the spasm.

Just at that very second the ambulance attendants from the Yorktown Volunteer EMS walked into the room behind me. I asked, "You don't have a defibrillator, do you?" Well, imagine Ray's fortune and my lucky relief. Yes, it was in their hands and being plugged in as I spoke. But at that moment no one realized just how lucky a situation it really was. In all the years of the existence of the Yorktown Ambulance Corps, this was the first defibrillator they had ever acquired. It had been donated that very afternoon and was being used for the first time three hours after the ambulance corps took possession of it. Just in time to shock Ray back into Yorktown. What a coincidence.

Years later, on the tenth anniversary of his "rebirth," Ray came into the office to thank me. I hadn't seen him for a couple of years, since I was just returning to practice in Yorktown after a two-year absence during which I ran for the U.S. Congress. We hugged and laughed, recalling our last encounter. As he was leaving, he told me that his wife, Gretyl, was in the car. She was too exhausted to come in, because she had been in the emergency room all night with chest pain.

I went out to the car to greet Gretyl. I remembered her as an attractive redhead with a pretty smile. This meeting was with an entirely different woman: tired, disheveled, and exhausted. Listening to her

Cardiac Warning Signs

We are in charge of our health. As such, we have to be on guard for signs and symptoms of cardiac disease—especially if there is a strong family history, if we suffer from hypertension or hyperlipidemia, if we smoke, have diabetes, or are sedentary. We cannot change our genes or heredity, but by eating properly, exercising regularly, and not smoking we can certainly forestall the onset of serious disease.

SIGNS & SYMPTOMS OF CARDIAC DISEASE:

- Extreme chest pain; unexplained jaw pain or shoulder pain
- Mild-to-moderate recurrent chest pain with exertion
- Mild unexplained chest pain with sweating
- General shortness of breath
- Shortness of breath or chest pain while walking up hills or stairs
- Shortness of breathe or chest pain while walking into the wind
- Unexplained swelling of your feet
- Unexplained cough

** One third of heart attacks in diabetics are **not** accompanied by chest pain.

** One third of heart attacks are **not** diagnosed in emergency rooms because their tests (EKG's, cardiac enzymes) come back as normal.

PRESCRIPTION:

- Get annual check ups which include an EKG, blood sugar and lipid profile.
- If you had a very suspicious event and your tests are normal, demand a stress test. Always get a nuclear stress test, as the regular non-nuclear testing misses about 25% of positive patients.
- Stress testing can be falsely positive and falsely negative; positive stress tests usually are followed by angiographic vascular studies.
- Many people have strongly positive family histories (example: father died of cardiac disease at age 45 or 50); these people should have bi-annual stress tests.

story, I insisted that she come inside the office because her symptoms were surely cardiac. In fact an EKG showed signs of a heart attack in progress. Ten years to the day of her husband's near demise, Gretyl was having a heart attack of her own. She too had to leave my office via an ambulance. This time, however, we didn't worry about the availability of a defibrillator.

• • •

Luck, or simply being in the right place at the right time, can almost be like having an invisible partner. But without the profit splitting and arguing over parking spaces. Even so, I cannot overemphasize—indeed I will not stop emphasizing—that we are each in charge of our own health and have to be on guard for signs and symptoms of disease. A preexisting family history of specific illnesses makes this even more of an imperative.

In each of the cases cited above, there were outwardly obvious indicators that something was terribly wrong. When the bishop came into my office, the change in appearance was striking and, though I hadn't seen him in a year, I can't imagine that the changes were any less obvious to those around him every day. Mark, the electronics store manager, nonchalantly told me not only that he had his hideously disturbing growth for over a year, *but that it was getting bigger and bigger!* Ray and Gretyl's cardiac conditions were painfully obvious (quite literally), yet Gretyl had already spent the night in the emergency room by the time our paths crossed. Think about what might have happened if I hadn't gone out to the car to greet her.

It is exceedingly rare that any of these conditions will "sneak up" on anyone. There are almost always early symptoms or high-risk behaviors that precede episodes such as these. So we have to stay on top of things. Get a physical each and every year, including blood tests, urine exams, stool exams for blood, mammograms and pap tests (for the ladies) and prostate exams (for the gents), and colonoscopies for those over the age of fifty—earlier if colon cancer runs in your family. Make sure you obtain copies of all of your lab results, cardiograms, X-rays, etc. Pay close attention not only to how you feel, but how you look—the tone of your skin, the tint of your eyes—and even how you smell. And if friends or family members make frequent comments to the effect of "you look like you could use some sun," or that you've lost a lot of weight when you haven't been trying to, you might want to consider what they're saying a little more closely.

Reaching Out

W E'RE ONLY A SHORT WAY THROUGH THE BOOK, but I'm sure that by now you've managed to pick up on one of my major messages: that the patient is just as responsible for health maintenance as the physician. Objectively this should be a no-brainer. Even the simplest animal possessed of the tiniest cranium instinctively knows to avoid doing things like eating poison plants, drinking tainted water, or asking a predator for spare change. But humans, unlike the lower animals, have been gifted with free will that can, and nearly always does, override some of the most basic instincts of self-preservation.

You will often hear physicians complain about patients who are not compliant with instructions. If you do not heed your doctor's advice, you assume this label. If you are told to take a certain pill but do not, you are non-compliant. Patients who smoke or who are overweight or who do not exercise? Non-compliant. Why? Because we told them to do otherwise, yet they keep on repeating behavior that has already brought them to the examination room and which is almost guaranteed to make their health deteriorate even further. Though far from funny, it's almost like watching a sitcom (which themselves are usually far from funny). After consulting with just such a patient recently, he answered his wife's question of, "What did the doctor tell you?" by saying, "The usual. Don't drink, don't smoke, and also I should lose weight." He had listened to my advice, but his noncommittal response foreshadowed the fact that he might not exactly heed it.

Though the Roman physician Galen enjoined his fellow healers to "first, do no harm," whether emotional or physical, you'll have to pardon me when I say that I feel physicians are entitled to call these folks names ("non-compliant" being the least offensive).

After years of saying the same thing, "Don't drink, don't smoke, lose weight," I finally learned that these words always fall on deaf ears. A fat person is fat not because they aspired to be fat, but because they didn't aspire *not* to be fat. And they probably have been on a thousand diets before they met me, and will probably be on a thousand more diets after we part ways. Same thing for my drinkers and

21

smokers; the comfort of doing what they've always done far out-weighs the cold, hard facts and solid advice they hear to the contrary in my office.

In fact, it usually takes a life event such as a heart attack or emergency surgery for them to return to "normal." Although for most patients it is a temporary return at best. They swear off cigarettes, pour out the cache of hidden booze, trim down, exercise, and eat properly. For a while, anyway. On average, the transformation usually lasts a year or so if it happens at all.

It's upsetting, at first, to see patients continue to do the same bad things over and over again, knowing that it will eventually get them as sure as driving on a bald tire will inevitably produce a nasty blowout. After years of experience, however, you eventually accept it as human nature. You continue to treat them, waiting for the other shoe to drop.

There are patients who even decide that they don't want to be treated for certain life-threatening diseases, such as cancer. Some just outright refuse the chance of survival by not taking chemotherapy. Of course, that's their right. If they still refuse treatment after I try to explain the benefits, I continue to take care of them without remorse or irritation.

I fully recognize that part of their unwillingness could be due to my "salesmanship," since all physicians are salesmen of a sort. And the pain and expense of certain therapies are admittedly a tough sell, even if the final transaction yields a new lease on life. Most of the time, however, there is either a deep-seated fear, honed since childhood, perhaps, after seeing a loved one suffer. Or perhaps it's just plain ignorance of the facts and an unwillingness to compromise their beliefs. "If it's my time to go, it's my time," many patients say to me. When, in fact, a simple mammogram or pap test or colonoscopy done routinely may detect diseases in their early and highly treatable stages, and thereby avoid needles, suffering, and premature death.

I have a relative who, because of fear, waited a year while suffering with daily rectal bleeding. Had she said something earlier, colonoscopic intervention would have found a small lesion, easily removable without surgery. In one year the lesion grew dangerously large and in the wrong place. Although she now wears a colostomy bag, fortunately, she is alive.

Comparison Table:
On Hearing and Being Heard

Possible Signs/Symptoms that Your Doctor Isn't Really Hearing You	Signs/Symptoms You're Not Telling Your Doctor Enough
• He doesn't make eye contact or is constantly distracted while you talk.	• You're doctor's asking you questions and you're not answering!
• She always discounts what you say with some variation of "It's all in your head."	• You know something you're not telling, because you think it's stupid, silly, selfish, 'out of left field', unimportant, or too personal.
• He casually tells you "Don't worry, everything is fine," when you sense deep-down that it might not be.	• You sense that there's more to say, but you can't put your finger on it.
• You feel intimidated and afraid to ask questions, express concerns, or make requests.	• Friends or family suggest things to ask or tell your doctor, but you brush it off.
• You walk out of the office feeling like you work for your doctor, instead of the other way around.	• When you're honest with yourself, you know you're just not fully committed to your health or healing process.
• You walk away feeling unheard.	

Woody Allen told the story years ago of when he started to suffer with headaches. Talk about fear of physicians, Woody was the epitome of fear. It also seems that he was quite reluctant to spend money. Anyway, the headaches eventually became intolerable and he was forced to see a doctor. After being examined, his physician informed him that he would need a few thousand dollars worth of testing. That was more then enough to send him running.

Then Woody remembered that his old friend Billy had suffered with similar headaches. So he called his long lost friend and Billy's mother answered. She informed him that Billy was dead. With that, Woody put down the phone. He immediately made appointments for all of the prescribed testing.

Two weeks and thousands of dollars later, he met with his physician and was relieved to learn that there was nothing seriously wrong. There were no brain tumors, no cancer. Excited, he called Billy's mother to apologize for his hasty phone call two weeks before and to say that he was sorry he had hung up on her. He explained that he had been upset because he had been suffering with the same headaches that had killed Billy. "Oh no," said the mother, "Billy got hit by a truck."

• • •

Getting back to my approach to noncompliant patients: I usually mention that I am sure that they've been on diets before and know the importance of taking better care of themselves, and that if I can help, I am there. Most patients respond by saying things like, "Yeah, I know I have to stop smoking and lose weight, but it's so hard," or "Doc, I don't want to take any medication; I don't even feel sick!" These failures to comply are not my responsibility, and I don't feel any sense of guilt or pique as I did when I first entered practice. Back then I blamed myself for not being able to get the message through. Years and years of witnessing the same mistakes by my patients have taught me that the patient has to assume responsibility for his health. I explain very carefully that if you have a stroke because you didn't take this medication for your blood pressure, that's your problem and that of your family and children. My job is to tell you what will happen to you if you don't comply with your prescribed treatment. I will still be here for you, but the guilt and the damage will be on your hands not mine. If they wind up in the hospital with an event, I never say, "I told you so." But I use the seriousness of the event as a reason to encourage full compliance.

This open and honest approach works most of the time in encouraging the patient to take her medication, maintain a more healthful diet, or increase physical activity. But I'll be darned if I can find a way to stop them from smoking.

There are those who suddenly change their habits without a life-threatening event. In lieu of a heart attack or other significant episode, sometimes some well-chosen words can work just as well. One of my other dearest friends, also named Don, but not the same don with the lower back problems from earlier, said he "woke up" when he said goodbye to the nurse after an exam. He said to her, quite casually, "I'll see you in a year."

She shot back, "What makes you think that you'll make it to next year?" At that very moment he had his epiphany.

If only we knew when that window of opportunity is open, when patients are ready to listen and get their epiphanies. I have yet to figure out the magic words to bring this state of revelation around for each and every person in need of it. Perhaps it is as simple as each of us asking ourselves, "What's in it for me?" If you take time to research what the future could hold if you keep on a destructive path and visualize what it would be like to live with the consequences—what it would be like to be so overweight that your activity and basic mobility are severely curtailed, or what it would be like to have your lungs so ravaged by smoking that a walk to the front door leaves you completely winded—maybe then you'll reach that tipping point where you finally realize the need to overwrite bad habits with good ones. Though we seem to be resistant to change by nature, the mind will always compel us toward pleasure and away from pain. The trick is to understand that pleasure in the short term could lead to less than pleasant consequences down the road. The time to change is now. Like my friend Don learned, there's no guarantee that you'll get another chance tomorrow.

Sometimes, though, it's neither the degrees on my walls nor the tone of my voice nor the diagnosis I've given that brings a patient around. Sometimes it's the strangest things that make people listen to a doctor.

I once had a sick patient who was known as the Red Canary. In case you're wondering (and I know you are), he got that name because he sold canaries that had a unique red hue to their feathers. At least, they did at the time he sold them. His secret for the red coloration was to feed his canaries paprika. After a while they turned red for him, long enough for him to make a sale, but lost their color after a few weeks at their new owners' homes.

Red was obviously an interesting character. We'd sit for a half hour or so and this thin, balding, elderly man would enthrall me with stories of his youth. He told me that, as a youngster, he kept a crow as a pet. Perhaps that is not terribly unusual in itself, but Red swore to me that the crow could talk as well as a parrot. I remember him telling me that the tongue of the crow had to be cut a certain way for it to speak. (I winced, wondering if those canaries knew how lucky they were to

simply ingest paprika to make them red, and not something more...
drastic.) Whether it's true or not, I don't know. But the story of him
raising a crow and ultimately letting it free only to have it hang around
his home for years, talking all the while, still brings a smile to my face.

One day, Red was in the hospital awaiting cancer surgery when,
during my rounds, he told me that he was going to refuse his life-saving surgery. When I asked him why, he said he was depressed. He
hadn't any money and had to depend upon his daughter and son-in-
law for everything. "Why," he murmured, "I don't even have any
money to turn on the TV service in my room."

Why one has to pay a hospital to watch TV in this day and age is
beyond me. In any event, I picked up the phone and ordered the TV
service and paid for it with my credit card. "Well Red," I said, "you
can't use not having TV service as an excuse for not having your
surgery anymore."

Red thought a minute and said, "Okay, I'll do it, doc."

• • •

Just as there are different "reasons" for a patient being non-compliant, there are different types of non-compliance. You can tell a
patient you've never even seen before that they need an "emergency
heart transplant," and they'll agree to step into an ambulance in a
heartbeat. Even if they don't have a cardiac symptom, and even if
they just came in for a cold. After all, the heart is a "vital organ."

And the mind? Well, that's another kind of "organ" altogether...

Tell a patient that they need to speak to a mental health expert
such as a psychologist or a psychiatrist, and they will disagree or try
to prove how wrong you are. "Why, doctor, you've only known me
fifteen minutes. How can you possibly think that in such a short period of time?" I'm often tempted to tell them that it was fourteen minutes more than I needed, but I usually don't. Most of these people can
be diagnosed by a layman in the street, that's how obvious their problem is. But for whatever reason, they'd prefer an immediate heart
transplant to an hour with a shrink.

My encounter with the "G" family exemplifies the denial often
associated with mental illness. Years ago I examined this young boy
for a school physical. He felt completely normal, and it was a surprise
for me to find his glands were swollen and his urine dark. The diag-

nosis of mononucleosis was obvious, with its associated hepatitis, even though the child felt fine.

I promptly called the father with my findings. He profusely thanked me and even sent a thank-you note for being such an "observant doctor." About two weeks later he sent his 18-year-old daughter, Debbie, in for a physical. Well, Debbie was certainly an attractive girl, but she just stared off into a corner of the room and didn't answer any question I asked. So we sat there together, and alone, for ten minutes, with neither of us speaking. Afterward, I called the father and said, "Mr. G., Debbie obviously has a severe mental problem and should be seen by someone right away." He had me put her on the phone and a few minutes later she left my office without a word.

After that, I didn't see her or anyone else in the family for about two years. Ultimately Debbie made her own new appointment. She had been hospitalized in various psychiatric institutions over the past year and a half and was now in a group home. She was also now able to communicate. When she came in for her appointment I was presented with a happy, energetic woman who might have been about the nicest person I had ever met.

You can't imagine how great a feeling it was to see her so warm and enthusiastic. She told me her father took her to another doctor after she left my office two years ago. The doctor screamed and yelled at her for not answering his questions and then threw her out of his office. Obviously the doctor had his own "issues" and couldn't deal with Debbie's. Debbie finally got her appropriate treatment six months later, but it sure wasn't because of her father—or my colleague.

Mental illnesses, especially depression, are interesting issues. Oftentimes I get new patients because their former physician, similar to the one I just described, has difficulties of his or her own. Often I hear from these dissatisfied patients that they themselves had recognized that they were feeling low or anxious. The response from their physicians? "I am a *medical* doctor; that's not my field." As if each doctor was a waitress who wouldn't bother to refill a customer's water glass because they weren't in "her section."

Technically that may be true, but sometimes just sitting down and showing concern and understanding—a little empathy never hurt—can set a patient on the right path. Another doctor's statement was "there's nothing wrong with you, just get a hold of yourself" and "you'll be alright." It's like the General George Patton situation, when he slapped a hospitalized soldier because the soldier had "shell shock" instead of recognizing that the mind can "freeze" someone forever.

Modern medicine has finally recognized the value of holistic healing and treating the patient as a unified whole—body, mind, and soul. The brain is just as vital an organ as the heart or any other; and while some minor injuries can be dealt with by "walking it off," that approach simply doesn't work if a person is unable to cope with what is going on in his or her own head.

• • •

Obviously the overall concept of mental health is a complicated one and is dependent on many factors that could be considered "intangibles" from a conventional, strictly medical perspective. Smoking, inactivity, substance abuse, all of these are concrete behaviors that have definite and proven effects on physical well-being. But as Debbie G's experience illustrates, the mind and spirit—as important to our health as the heart and lungs—are unfamiliar territory to many physicians, often of secondary importance to the more easily identifiable and quantifiable afflictions of the physical body. As the holistic, whole organism–approach gains wider currency in the world of medicine, I am often shocked to find that some of my colleagues still fail to address the impact of non-physical difficulties; especially because of the universality of some of these situations, which guarantees that even physicians themselves have a high chance of gaining first-hand experience with them.

For instance, just as important as remaining physically active or observing a healthy diet is the need to have and maintain a sense of purpose in life, to have direction and feel somehow useful and worthwhile. Some of the biggest challenges to the sense of self-worth come with the life-changing events of retirement and divorce.

MATTERS PSYCHOLOGICAL/MENTAL

DIAGNOSIS:

Clearly, the "no pain, no gain" philosophy works about as well in a hospital setting as it does on the playing field. Patients can't just "walk it off" when they're unable to cope with the messages their own minds are sending.

All doctors specialize, but our oath is absolute. If it is in our power to heal, we should try to heal body, mind, and soul. In the great restaurant of modern medicine, every patient is sitting in our "section."

Signs / Symptoms that Your Problem Might Need More than Just a Pill:

- You feel sad, angry, or depressed for a prolonged period of time.
- You feel excessive fear, worry, or anxiety.
- You have consistent "dark thoughts" or confused thinking.
- You experience extreme highs and lows in your mood.
- There are dramatic changes in your eating or sleeping habits.
- Your life feels dull, listless, and meaningless.
- You feel withdrawn, isolated, unable or unwilling to connect with others.
- You're having hallucinations or delusions.
- You're having an increasingly difficult time dealing with daily issues.
- You're suffering from many unexplained physical maladies.
- Your one drink to relax at night has turned into several… and starts earlier.
- You don't want to get out of bed—ever again.

PRESCRIPTION:

- Don't just tell yourself, "I'm fine," and leave it at that. Denial is not a river in Egypt, it's a dangerous game where we rationalize (rational lies) our life away.
- Don't listen to anyone else who just tells you you're fine; most people are uncomfortable with real emotion and crisis because it reflects back to them their own hidden demons and unresolved issues.
- Keep a journal about your life and your issues, and see if you can gain some insight. Sometimes just writing about your thoughts, feelings, and concerns can create a cathartic experience that clears away a lot of the mental and emotional debris—at least enough so that you can see what's *really* going on.
- If you have a spiritual practice, use it. Prayer and meditation can be a powerful process of reconnecting to your core sense of peace, passion, and purpose.
- If you have a friend or family member who can listen without judgment, try talking it out. Sometimes just being heard and seen

is all the healing you need; and often when we talk out loud, we hear and see *ourselves* more clearly.

- Take a class, seminar, or read a book about the subject you're struggling with, if you know what it is. The power to heal yourself is within you, sometimes you just need a few tools for the do-it-yourself job.

- If you know the source of mental and emotional stress, someone or something at work or home, perhaps, take actions to deal with it. If it's a physically abusive situation, seek outside help immediately.

- If all of the above fails, or if you are having suicidal thoughts or are unable to function in everyday life, immediately seek professional help.

PROGNOSIS

We all have the ability to be our own physicians; or at least our own diagnosticians. The powers of the mind, body, and spirit to heal itself are far beyond what we have yet discovered. If you are willing to trust your innate power, acknowledge your real state of mind and emotions, and do whatever you must to heal your broken heart, aching soul, mental issues, or chemical imbalances, you will not only get to "know thyself," but you will greatly increase your ability to "heal thyself" as well.

Retirement is often terribly unhealthy. How often have people lived and worked toward the goal of retirement, stating they will keep their traveling plans on hold until their so-called "golden years"? And how often have you heard about someone setting their sights on such a goal, only to die within a year of reaching that goal? They worked relentlessly to retire, planning for a great second lifetime of travel, learning, and experience, only to lost the opportunity to enjoy those golden years because all too often they get sick and die before that magical time arrives. It is a well-documented fact that many elderly people die shortly after a life event such as the marriage or graduation of a grandchild or great grandchild. "Grandma looked forward to that wedding for six months, then died two days later." I've heard many similar stories during my career. Having reached the anticipated event, they then give in to the disease inside. For too many, retirement itself seems to be that goal and, once reached, a person can see the flat line of the future stretch out before them. Rather than the "permanent vacation" they expected it to be, many come to see life after retirement as an empty landscape with nothing to compel them forward, a time that is spent dealing with the "inevitable" decline of the body. An unfortunate number of retired folks become less social, withdrawn, inactive, fatter and less in shape the notorious couch potato that just sits around all day and watches TV.

It may be human nature, but it's far from natural.

There are so many positive benefits to maintaining some sort of activity or avocation after retirement. Perhaps not at the same tempo as before, but something that keeps the body and mind engaged. A regular level of social interaction with colleagues and the public is important to being part of an interactive society. It gives you a reason for getting up in the morning.

Though not retired, I took two years away from practicing medicine to make an (unfortunately) unsuccessful run for Congress. As a working family physician, my days were filled with telephone conferences with colleagues as we compared diagnoses, discussed patients and journal articles, remarked on current trends inside and outside medicine, and even dished about friends. Our consultations with each other were equal parts work and socialization. When my campaign was over and I had been away from medicine for some time, I noticed a drastic change in the quality of my interaction with my fellow healers. They had stopped calling me somewhere along the way, and when I reached out to them the dynamic was different. It felt almost as if I had been removed from the social/professional "body" of which I had been a part, and that the space I had once occupied had since healed over, leaving me no place to which I could easily return. All of my retired medical friends related similar experiences as their retirement forced upon them the necessity of developing a whole new set of friends.

People need to feel useful, especially the elderly. As aging sets in and one's physical strength lessens, many of us lose our independence and begin a slide into a sort of existential despair. We feel helpless, useless, and irrelevant, and our physical bodies begin to succumb to this negative outlook. As one simple tool to combat this, I always encourage people with elderly parents to ask small favors from them in the course of a normal day—please watch the children for an hour, please help me paint this wall, etc. Or suggest a type of exchange of favors to lessen the sense of dependency they may feel. If, for example, an older relative needs a ride to their doctor's office for an appointment, propose that you'll drive, but could they please give you a hand with cooking for the kids, helping in the garden, walking the dog. This turns the whole thing around, as now you are asking them to "pay" or "work" for something and thereby giving them a sense of value and self-confidence.

Most of us are living longer and healthier these days, so the need to have some sort of *raison d'être* even after our professional lives come to a close is especially acute. As proof of the effectiveness of this approach I can offer no better example than that of the Rolling Stones. With an average age of 64.3 years for the remaining original members involved in their two-year long *Bigger Bang* tour, the Stones easily qualify as active seniors. And if Keith Richards can still muster the strength to perform after his laundry list of substance abuse problems, there's no reason for you to let arthritis or the need for bifocals get in your way.

• • •

Another window into the importance of usefulness for both physical and mental health is divorce and its effects on the principals involved. In addition to the more obvious emotional ups and downs of the process, the attendant financial strains, and, all too often, the suffering children, there is for many the unforeseen and unpleasant necessity of having to redefine and reevaluate the very purpose and direction of their lives.

There is a phrase that former Israeli Prime Minister Shimon Peres once used when talking about the lasting effects of Israel's capture of the West Bank in 1967. He explained that once you take two eggs and scramble them, you can never go back and make the scrambled egg into the original form. As fundamentally true as those words may be, our natural resistance to swift and drastic change make them especially unpalatable and difficult to integrate for someone going through a less-than-amicable divorce. Indeed, the process of dismantling a marriage and the life that two people have tried to build together can bring out the worst in a person. Sometimes that behavior is directed at the erstwhile partner in the form of false claims of spousal or child abuse, something to gain the upper hand in legal proceedings or to simply dish out some emotional payback. Some, consumed by feelings of anger and betrayal, go the extra step and take action against their ex's property or even person. One of my regular patients had to have an order of protection taken out against her ex-husband after suffering through frightening threats and acts of intimidation. In another case, a divorced couple, each of whom chose to remain in my care after their separation, somehow managed to schedule back-to-back appointments with my office on the same day. What followed was a mad dash by my staff and myself to keep them in separate wings of the building and unaware of each other's presence, lest an ugly and potentially explosive situation ensue (mission accomplished, you'll be happy to know).

Others turn their misery inward and undo themselves. I don't mean to be unnecessarily flip or melodramatic, but high levels of stress such as can be caused by divorce are like the match touched to the fuse of a string of potential maladies. Perhaps in an effort to keep up and maintain control you'll let your diet lapse, court weight gain, smoke or drink more, and proceed down the path to diabetes, high blood pressure, and a nearly endless list of other conditions. Perhaps the most compelling case I've ever personally witnessed was that of "Tom," a patient of mine who went into a literal tailspin of depression after his divorce and the loss of custody of his children. In short order he developed a debilitation drug problem that caused him to eventually lose his job and further curtailed the contact he was allowed to have with his kids.

Incidentally, and call me old-fashioned if you must, I find it particularly heartbreaking when women fall victim to this syndrome. In my role as family physician, I can't tell you how many women I've seen fall into the trap of becoming dependent on a husband only to end up divorced, alone, saddled with children and a host of other responsibilities that end up thrust upon her and her alone. This, and the fact that I am the father of two daughters, is why I'm a big advocate of the idea that a woman should study, develop a career, and explore the world on her own before even entertaining the idea of marriage. But that's a topic for another book.

It would be wise to add here that there are entire industries that reap huge revenues from our weaknesses and vulnerabilities. In any given year, according to the National Institute of Mental Health, nearly ten percent of the population suffers from some sort of depression.

In a bid to cope, many of these will turn to therapists, either psychologists or licensed social workers, or psychiatrists who increasingly recommend or prescribe what has become a veritable rainbow of pharmaceutical remedies. I discount neither the usefulness of psychotherapy and psychiatry, nor the effectiveness of pharmaceuticals in general in treating certain conditions and certain patients. Still, it is impossible to deny that sometimes some individuals become addicted to therapy and/or dependent on prescription medication while mistakenly believing that they are tackling the obstacles that lay before them. Getting past an "event" and moving on with your life is not characterized by constantly rehashing and dwelling on things past, whether it's to your shrink or to your friends and family, or by popping a pill to calm nerves frayed by unresolved anxieties that are carelessly characterized as ongoing disorders.

What I am trying to say with these stories and observations is that part of striving for and maintaining good health is knowing how to enjoy our lives, no matter what. Life, as they say, is for living, and a life-changing event like divorce or retirement in no way lessens the unique value of your life and your contribution to the human race. What's done is done, and can not be undone, and the future is yet unwritten. No matter how many eggs have been scrambled, there is always a new one waiting to be hatched in each and every life. If you deal head-on with your problems, let go of the past, and focus on living, you'll not only create a new story, you'll become a hero in the adventure of your life.

And don't worry—there will always be plenty of people available to help keep therapists and drug companies solvent.

Some People We Meet
Along the Way

Aヵ LARGE PART OF BEING HUMAN INVOLVES interaction with other humans. It's an inherent part of our collective nature, and it's how we as a species have managed to come as far as we have.

Obviously a medical practitioner gets to interact with a lot of people from countless backgrounds and professions; prince or pauper, male or female, Black, White, or otherwise, everyone needs to visit a doctor at some point in their lives, whether they want to or not. But in my case luck, fate, and an outgoing nature have enabled me to log some fascinating interpersonal experiences over the course of my career. In sharing them with you, I'd like to think that I bring the topic of this section full circle by sharing not only tales reflecting a doctor's humanity, but the rainbow of people that make up our world. Whether stars or on skid row, it was in the doctor's office that our paths crossed, underscoring a valuable lesson that I hope I have thus far managed to communicate.

• • •

During my residency, I became friendly with an older alumnus of New York Medical College, Benjamin Gilbert. Dr. Gilbert was quite famous because, at the time, he was the one and only Theater Doctor.

He had worked his way through medical school playing drums in bands on and around Broadway, and saw no reason to cut his association with the world of performance and performers once he got his degree. He opened his practice in a hotel on 45th Street , a sleazy place, but with the raffish air of the demimonde of the theater. Anyone who got sick in the Broadway district, be they famous or just a theatergoer, called his number, and for years his name was in every *Playbill* printed, listed simply as "The Theater Doctor." By the time of my residency he had his foot in every restaurant and hotel along that Great White Way, becoming so busy that he regularly hired New York Medical College residents to help him out. So on my free evenings twice a week I would moonlight, sitting in his office on 45th Street awaiting some of the most interesting calls from theaters and hotels.

One evening a fellow resident and I were called to the famous Latin Quarter night club. Though New York City is still known for both the number and quality of its nightlife spots, there is currently nothing that can compare with the old Latin Quarter for glitz and glamour. Aside from their well-deserved reputation for dispensing the best in food, drink, dancing, and entertainment to its patrons, they were also known for their revolving chorus line of statuesque showgirls, shimmying and high-kicking in costumes that would still qualify as risqué, even in this current era of exposed flesh as the norm. That evening, all eight showgirls developed an allergic reaction to some kind of paint or dye they had put on their breasts as part of their costumes. The cure: cortisone cream, applied topically.

They had just started making cortisone at the time, and we could only get our hands on one tube. It was enough to treat our bewitching group of patients, but it meant that it limited our options to just one of us treating just one woman at a time. So we came to a just and equitable distribution of labor (what with there only being one tube of cortisone), and proceeded to work our way down a line of beautiful women, applying the cortisone first to one breast, then to the other breast, and repeated the procedure four times apiece. My colleague and I always remembered the night the show could go on because of us. (After all, how could we forget?)

More often, though, my work for the Theater Doctor involved tending to a reveler or theatergoer who had suddenly fallen ill or managed to overindulge in one vice or another. And of course, the "ladies of the night" would begin to stop by at around 5:00 A.M., roughly the end of their "shift," with their run of the mill complaints of colds, sore throats, and the like. I was more likely to deal with that sort of talent than the type that made their livings inside the theaters. But every once in a while, something would happen on my watch that would, for a few moments, propel me to the A-list.

One evening, Pearl Bailey was playing on Broadway and couldn't go on because she had lost her voice. It was only a short time to curtain, and an immediate call went out to Dr. Gilbert's office. The Theater Doctor had a "special" throat spray for such situations; as one of his assistants on call that evening, I had to run it over to the theater and treat Ms. Bailey. While the show was being held up, I was backstage spraying ground-up aspirin through a nebulizer straight into her throat. The show started a half-hour late, but Pearl could now sing.

• • •

During this time, I began studying Tae Kwon Do. A beginning medical professional is subject to a grueling schedule, from the first day of training right on through residency and often beyond. It is easy to fall into a rut or become overwhelmed with the amount of work involved, and I thought Tae Kwon Do offered both healthy exercise as well as a healthy outlet for any frustrations I might have had. My sparring mate was an up-and-coming dancer by the name of Gregory Hines. Because of his long legs and what seemed to be a gift for dance, Greg was a martial arts natural. Once he kicked me in the chest so hard during a workout that I couldn't take a deep breath for a month. We soon became good friends, and I later became his and his first wife's physician.

My wife at the time had never before been backstage, so I asked Greg if we could stop by after one of his Broadway shows. As it turned out, the reality was much less glamorous than what she had imagined, and she was confronted with a drafty and cavernous backstage area where the dressing room was up several flights of creaky stairs and filled with a squadron of male dancers in various states of undress rushing to get out of costume and makeup and just go home.

The next morning Greg called to ask for some help, saying he was sick and thought he had a fever. I asked how high his fever was, but he told me he didn't have a thermometer, so I asked him to take his pulse. As he did so, I explained to him that Hippocrates, way back in 400 B.C., was able to determine that someone suffering from a fever develops an increased heart rate, and that every extra ten points of one's pulse equals a one-degree rise in ones' body temperature. So if the average normal pulse is 70-80, and the pulse during illness is 100, the temperature should be 2 or 3 degrees higher than 98.6, or 100 to 101 degrees.

By the time we finished the mathematical quiz, I had diagnosed Greg as having a mild cold and told him to buy a thermometer.

• • •

My nature as a "people person" has not only earned me friendships with religious prelates, Broadway stars, and semi-nude showgirls. In a happy and gratifying coincidence, it also led to me being knighted by the Italian government.

The whole thing started as a favor to a Roman friend, Aldo. His next-door neighbor's daughter had an upper eyelid deformity called *chapeau de gendarme* (so named because of its resemblance to a French policeman's rounded hat). Did I know of anyone in the States that could repair such a distorted lid? When I got back to the States I researched and found the man who was the leading authority in treating this problem I had never heard of. I related the situation and the doctor gave me the contact information of a former student of his in London. I forwarded the information and heard two months later that the lid was successfully repaired in England.

After that, a slow but steady stream of requests and queries began to come in from friends and neighbors of this girl's family. Some of these involved diseases I was utterly unfamiliar with, like massive abnormal serpentine venous malformation, and/or required intricate surgery to correct them. There were patients with rare tumors and seemingly incurable cancers who wrote and sent their medical records and hopes.

I decided that Italy had helped me become a physician, so the least I could do was repay them. There are many fine physicians in Italy, serving a population of 50 million Italians. But with our population at over 250 million we see many more rare diseases, and some of our research centers are the best in the world. So I started translating each record received and forwarded it to the best specialists I could find, then forwarded their treatment recommendations and observations back to the Italian families. After a few years, people wrote directly to the Italian Consulate in New York City asking them to forward their records to the Dr. Klein who helped their friend or relative. After approximately 1,000 patients, I received a call from the Italian Consul General saying that he was recommending me for governmental honors because of my work on behalf of my Italian "patients." I thought the whole thing was truly exciting because no one in my family was ever so honored, but I knew that these things were always lost in seas of red tape and were constantly at the mercy of whatever government official was in charge of such matters. Besides, one does these things for the feeling of doing something to help someone in need, not necessarily for accolades. So I filed the idea in the back of my mind and went about my business treating people in Westchester and helping those Italians I could.

About three years later, the Consulate in New York called to say they were visited by an Italian citizen who had just gotten off an Alitalia plane from Sicily looking for the doctor from New York who had helped his neighbor. The man, Luigi, spoke no English and flew alone, without much for money, and told his story to a Hispanic Alitalia baggage handler at J.F.K. Airport, the only person he could find who understood him. The baggage man was so moved that he invited Luigi to stay at his Queens apartment with him and his wife at no cost. After depositing his bags at the Queens apartment, Luigi took a train to the Consulate.

His son, Luigi told the Consul's staff, could only move on his tippy toes, and then only for some short distance before he fell to the ground. He was told by his Sicilian doctor that the boy had been born with "half a brain" (that's what Luigi said; I don't know how true that assessment was, but Luigi did have an x-ray of the child's skull, which was normal). Many corrective operations for this abnormality were proposed, but none helped. "If they could fly to the moon," Luigi asked, "why can't they help my son walk?" But then he heard of a doctor in the United States who could possibly help, and he came directly to New York.

Luigi brought a video of his son, which I brought to a friend who ran the special hospital for children in Valhalla, New York, known as Blythedale. After viewing the tape, his staff neurologist told me that the child had cerebral palsy. I remembered that one of my patients, Janet, had a daughter, Elyse, who suffered with cerebral palsy and was paralyzed. She went to a specialized school at St. Agnes Hospital in White Plains. To my surprise, the physician who ran the program was a woman from Rome, Dr. Picci. I had a car take Luigi to St. Agnes.

He met Janet and Elyse. He met the Italian physician and he saw twenty or thirty children who suffered with the same disease as his son. The gratifying outcome was that the director of the program knew of a very similar program in Rome, and Luigi's son is now enrolled in that program. The boy will never walk properly, but he is at least in the hands of caring and trained people.

Shortly thereafter, I was visiting in Rome when my office called to say that they received a letter from the office of President of Italy informing them that I was awarded the honor of *Cavilliere* (knight) of the State of Italy for meritorious work for its citizens. Though it took nearly four years and two government administrations, I was still filled with gratitude that the Italian government should see fit to acknowledge my work. It is an honor not so easily bestowed on non-Italian, nor non-Italian American, foreigners. *Grazie.*

• • •

Just after my run for Congress, I worked for six months in Key Biscayne, Florida. One day, this man walked unannounced into the private office of the physician for whom I was filling in. He had short, grayish blond, wind blown hair, the well-chewed nub of a lit cigar dangling from his lips, and a series of ugly bruises around his head. He looked exactly like a hard-aged sixty year old, but he happened to be wearing a dress with no make-up, wig, or any other attempt at feminization; she was a man simply wearing a woman's dress. I honestly didn't know whether someone was playing a joke on me. It wasn't April Fools' or Halloween. "What's with this?" I thought.

"Name's Gloria," he said in a husky voice.

My short silence was interrupted by the nurse, who followed "Gloria" into the room carrying her chart. "This is Gregory Hemingway, son of the late Ernest Hemingway," she said, as if that would explain everything.

During my intake discussion with Gloria/Gregory (the medical essentials of which I have since forgotten), I learned about both the Hemingway family and the tragedies that befell many members (so many suicides), as well as her own troubled history, as Gloria billowed smoke around the room from the still lit cigar (though I have trouble with smoking, Hemingway was cigar buddies with the doctor I was temporarily replacing). As Gregory, he fathered eight children and had been a physician in Montana, but lost his license years before because of alcohol and his demons. Having returned to his father's legendary stomping grounds with a new identity, she was constantly getting into brawls with police and had a long arrest record. All of these facts were nonchalantly offered.

There was irony in what was an obvious incongruity. While Ernest portrayed the life of a "he-man"—hunting, fighting, embarking on adventure—his son Gregory, despite the brawling, was going out of his way to present the opposite end of the spectrum. Or at least he tried. It occurred to me later that Gregory's brawling and alcoholism was not much different from his father's behavior.

• • •

As a physician, I am called upon to care for many types of people, and for some I have developed a deep dislike, such as ones who are addicts or criminals. While training as an intern, I had to learn the lessons of trying to care for alcoholics, who are just another type of addict, despite my personal feelings. After devoting hours and hours expending physical, mental, and emotional energy, I have been sorely let down by patients who promise to quit after weeks of detox in the hospital, yet end up returning for the same detox just weeks after their previous hospitalization. These are just patients, not family, yet the emotional let down can be hurtful.

I'm reminded of Pam, a patient, whose father was the editor of a famous weekly family magazine. For years, he would regularly check himself into a hotel on Friday night and binge on alcohol straight through until Monday morning. He would then call his wife, who just as regularly dutifully rescued him by rushing to wherever he was and sobering and dressing him for work. After several years of this, she wisely stopped and the father then dragged Pam into the same roll. She did this for six months and then came to see me. She was distraught because of her new roll, which was now impacting on her children and husband as well. The answer was obvious and we discussed it. Regardless of her love for and devotion to her father, she did him no good by being his enabler. Her mother had managed to figure out that lesson, now it was Pam's turn to accept it.

Although, as the saying goes, it can "take a village" of compassion to help those who have taken a stumble along the way, it also takes endurance and courage, particularly when dealing with a drug or alcohol addict. All too often the urge to help, to heal, and too protect is co-opted by the addict's ability to manipulate these instincts to turn the helper into the enabler. I make this aside after these stories of Gloria and Pam because my years in general practice have demonstrated for me the near-epidemic proportions of the problem of substance abuse in America today. With this in mind, I'm including on the following pages a table of signs and symptoms that are nearly always indicative of some type of substance abuse or related emotional problem, as well as a list of resources for those who, for one reason or another, must deal with addicts in and out of recovery.

• • •

It's not just tales of heartbreak and big names that make for good anecdotes. There were certainly a number of episodes that more than a small element of comedy to them. One elderly patient of mine, who also happens to be a cousin of mine, told me that he one day began to experience chest pains. Fearing he was suffering some sort of cardiac episode, he was faced not only with the terror of a heart attack, but with the near paralysis of indecision that so often overcomes so many of us in emergency situations. So, not sure what was happening or what to do, Milton came to the decision that if he played some basketball, he would get a better handle on the situation. If it was really a heart attack, his reasoning went, the exertion would force his heart problem to "show itself;" if there was nothing wrong, at least he would get some exercise and perhaps fend off any future heart problems. (As if it was so easy!) Fortunately, Milton didn't have a heart problem.

Unfortunately, Benny did. Benny was a real character—a Bronx native with the accent to prove it, he was a locally-known bookmaker who made no secret of his numerous and far-reaching "connections" with various "legitimate businessmen." He came into my office one day complaining of a sore throat. I examined him, diagnosed him, and was prepared to send him on his way in under ten minutes, when he turned to me as he was leaving the examination room and asked in that classic accent, "Hey doc, how come I got dis pain in my chest when I lifted da gobbige cans dis mornin'?" His new and completely unexpected complaint gave me pause, and I insisted he stay a bit longer while I did an electrocardiogram. The EKG revealed that Benny was, in fact, having a heart attack, and I immediately sent for an ambulance to take him from my office to the hospital.

That night I made a quick stop into the hospital to check up on Benny, and when I got there I found him surrounded by three or four men wearing expensive track suits and awash in jewelry. They all stopped their conversation as I walked in, and swiveled their heads to follow my actions as I examined Benny's charts and tried to gauge

Signs & Symptoms of Drug and Alcohol Addiction:

- Severe loss of appetite, change in eating habits, frequent nausea or vomiting
- Bloodshot or watery eyes, or dilated pupils
- Frequent colds, runny nose, dizzy spells, fatigue, shaky hands, and noticeable loss of motor coordination
- Slurred or unusually rapid speech
- Mood swings (virtually all mood-altering drugs produce swings from euphoria to depression; an abuser may swing from passivity to anger)
- Personality changes, defensiveness, blaming others, or feeling victimized
- Strained communication; unwillingness to discuss important issues
- Withdrawal from family activities
- Change in dress and friends; sudden deterioration of long relationships
- Lack of self discipline; inability to follow rules or complete homework or work-related duties
- Apathy—little or no interest in meaningful activities
- Anxious behavior; seemingly chronic jittery, jerky, or uneven movements

PRESCRIPTION OF RESOURCES AND REFERRALS:

- Adult Children of Alcoholics: 310-534-1815
- Al-Anon/Alateen Family Groups: 888-4-AL-ANON
- Alcohol Treatment Referral Hotline: 800-252-6465
- Alcoholics Anonymous: 212-870-3400
- Chemically Dependent Anonymous: 202-966-9115
- Child Help USA: 800-222-4453
- Cocaine Anonymous: 310-559-5833
- Families Anonymous: 800-736-9805
- Girls and Boys Town National Hotline: 800-448-3000
- Marijuana Anonymous: 800-766-6779
- Methadone Anonymous: www.methadone-anonymous.org/
- Nar-Anon Family Groups: 800-477-6291

- National Alliance on Mental Illness (NAMI): 703-524-7600
- National Center for Victims of Crime: 800-211-7996
- National Domestic Violence Hotline: 800-787-3224
- National Suicide Prevention Lifeline: 800-273-8255
- Secular Organizations for Sobriety: 310-821-8430
- Self Help and Information Exchange (SHINE): 570-961-1234
- Self Management and Recovery Training (SMART Recovery): 866-951-5357
- Women for Sobriety: 215-536-8026

how he was coming along, which was amazing when you consider the fact they didn't have a neck between the lot of them. I wasn't sure whether to be intimidated by the presence of these men who fairly radiated a sense of menace, or to laugh at the fact that I had somehow fallen into an outtake reel from one of the *Godfather* movies. In an effort to break the tension, I opted to err on the side of comedy ... or so I thought. I put on my most earnest face as I walked over to the large, square cardiac monitor—the type we used back in those days— that was covered with green hospital fabric and pinned to Benny's pajama shirt, and said to the assembly, "Be careful, that thing is a tape recorder." Though I thought I was taking steps to ease the mood in the room, the gentlemen evidently took me at my word; their faces went from wearing expressions of somewhat menacing detachment to showing a quick succession of emotions and thoughts. Was this whole thing a set-up? Is Benny in on it? Can we toss this doctor guy out the window and still make it out of here?

Laughter may sometimes be the best medicine, but it was obviously contraindicated in this case. Quickly reading the situation, I piped in with, "Only kidding." Finally, the tension level cooled enough for the bunch of us to enjoy a bit of a laugh, but I made a note to remain on my toes around any of Benny's future business associates.

• • •

For another one-time patient of mine, the problem was neither indecision nor ignorance of her condition, but how to properly get the most effective treatment for her problem. This was some forty years ago during my internship at Metropolitan Hospital on the east side of

Manhattan, when a woman who we would now describe as a bag lady came to our emergency room and presented with a very general complaint of vaginal pain. She responded in the negative when asked if she had been the victim of a rape or other violence, had no symptoms that would have indicated a sexually transmitted disease, and was evasive with all other questions. She just complained mightily of a pain inside her and kept pushing me to do an internal pelvic exam. Not wanting to turn away a genuinely sick woman, I acquiesced, put on my gloves, and put her in the stirrups. Within seconds of beginning the exam, I found a ten-dollar bill folded over on itself several times and inserted deep inside the vaginal canal. As soon as I extracted the note and presented her with my findings, her demeanor suddenly brightened as she began to thank me profusely. She then explained to me that because she regularly slept on the streets, she had to hide her money in a secure location. Unfortunately, she had gone so far in trying to put her cash out of reach that she herself could not retrieve the bill.

• • •

Whether or not you find the above stories funny in any way has a lot to do with your personal sense of morality, of propriety, your ability to empathize, and a host of other variables. While I might find what I consider to be a harmless source of levity in some aspects of my job, many readers may be shocked to find a doctor being so seemingly flip about the ailing, the weak, women, or ethnic stereotypes.

But regardless of your personal feelings, laughter really can be the best medicine. And if not the best, it certainly can't hurt. Life presents us with serious challenges and more than enough to worry about every day—war, taxes, illness, and other mundane dramas of everyday life. Approaching such questions with a dose of humor doesn't demean the seriousness of life, it makes it more palatable. A teaspoon of humor will not only help the medicine go down, it will put a smile on your face, a spring in your step, and help lift your spirits above any given situation.

PART 2

PLACES

Introduction

AS MUCH AS I'VE LEARNED FROM MY PATIENTS and about myself through my time in medicine, I've also learned from the places medicine has taken me. I'm not just talking about my schooling in Rome or my work in Israel or my service in the navy and marines, although all of these experiences had profound, wonderful effects on my life.

I'm also talking about the journeys of the spirit I've been able to take, the journeys of the heart and mind, of learning and experience. My journeys have enabled me to not only learn new languages, new social customs, and which fork to use for which course. In addition, they have taught me how to be humble, how to be empathetic, and how to see things through the eyes of others, as much as such a thing is really possible.

More importantly, my journeys have taught me why all of these lessons were worth learning. And in this section, I'd like to share some of them with you. There are certain defining characteristics in life that seem to simultaneously link us and divide us, as we adher to different cultures and faiths, the different things we value at different times. If approached correctly, the journey through life shows us that these things transcend the very boundaries we impose on them, doing more to link us that keep us apart.

Life has been compared to everything from a marathon to a dream to a box of chocolates. I prefer to think of life as being like a train, each milestone and watershed experience being like a station on the trip. This train keeps going, rain or shine, and never stops until the ultimate stop. During the journey, passengers board and disembark at the many different stations along the way. The more people we meet, and the more stations we pass through, the more knowledge we obtain.

Prepare for the Journey

I'M NOT THE ONLY DOCTOR WITH A LOT OF STORIES. The practice of medicine lends itself easily to anecdotes that can shock and/or entertain. It must have something to do with the intersection of fear, helplessness, and semi-public nudity that we encounter on a regular basis. I like to think that my stories, however, have a little extra something, a little more "oomph." I firmly believe that this is because I've managed to take a different road through life than most of my peers, particularly with regards to my path through the medical profession.

In contrast to the most widely held image of the physician (particularly the Jewish physician from New York), my route to becoming a doctor began as an enlistee—first with the Navy, then the Marine Corps—assigned to the duties of hospital corpsman. From there I developed the drive, skill, and great good fortune to be able to attend medical school in Rome, Italy. The years spent in the Eternal City introduced me to many wonderful things I may not have otherwise experienced, and created in me an inquisitive nature that has allowed me to continue learning and experiencing via my love for travel and discovery, my appreciation for diverse cultures, and my long-standing love affair with the land where it all started.

My time in Italy also gave me my first real window into the mechanics of how cultures differ from each other in the treatment of maladies as well as people. For instance, it was in Italy that I was introduced to what the locals call *mal di fegato*. Literally translatable as "badness of the liver," it is the Italian manifestation of a belief that stretches back through time and across the globe: that our health and our behavior are dictated by the relative balance of four specific bodily fluids or glandular secretions that were once known as "humors." Each of these substances controlled a certain temperament which, in turn, was governed by the organ or gland or membrane that the ancients most closely associated with that humor. So if, say, you were a mild-mannered, church-going, everyday artisan in the 16th century who suddenly became grouchy after taking ill, the village doctor—who doubled as the village barber and was often the village alchemist, as well—would diagnose you as having a surfeit of yellow bile, obviously caused by an overactive gall bladder. He would then prescribe some course of treatment that was equal parts excruciating and ineffective, perhaps something involving leeches or human feces[2], but which constituted marked improvements over the previously standard "witchcraft" diagnosis and "burning-at-the-stake" prescription.

Under this system of thought, the liver is thought to govern the blood, which controls a person's optimism, cheer, and sense of self-confidence (consider the definition of the word *sanguine,* which was originally the term used to describe a patient suffering from an overactive or inflamed liver). Though these are all crucial qualities to anyone's well-being, it was widely believed that these minor ailments of the liver were easy to treat because blood was the most easily and consistently accessible of the humors; after all, it was and is no great feat to get a patient to bleed a bit. Even so, as the popularity of bleeding as a medical procedure waned, the belief has persisted in many parts of Europe and Asia that many garden variety illnesses are caused by a simple malfunctioning of the liver—constipation, headaches, indigestion and heartburn, fatigue—and can be treated with "liver medicines" that have their roots in the folk pharmacopeia and old-wives' tales, but which are now mass produced by European drug companies.

Despite the images many Americans once had of the naturally urbane and cosmopolitan European, it is truly amazing how popular and pervasive this belief remains. Some years ago, I found myself on an Alitalia flight to Rome when a flight attendant ("stewardess" at the time) got on the public address and asked if a doctor was on-board to tend to an ill passenger. I volunteered my services and the attendant led me toward the patient. As luck would have it, a former med school classmate of mine was on the same plane and had also come to the patient's aid. The young man we had come to help was complaining of tightness in his chest and swelling around his mouth, and we quickly realized that he was having an allergic reaction to the shrimp that was served for lunch.

---

2   The "natural philosopher" Robert Boyle had a recipe for an allegedly soothing eye lotion that involved taking human feces "of a good Colour and Consistence" and drying it until it can be reduced to powder, which is then to be "blown once, twice or thrice a Day, as occasion shall require, into the Patient's Eyes." This is the same man who gave us the principle in chemistry known as "Boyle's Law."

This is generally an easy situation to manage with simple drugs like epinephrine, Benadryl, or steroids to combat the histamines that cause irritation of mucous membranes and airway constriction during an allergic reaction. But when my colleague and I asked the attendant for the emergency medical bag that we had assumed would be on the plane in anticipation of just such an emergency, we were both shocked and dismayed to find that it was full of vials of "liver extract," "liver supplements," injectable vitamin B-12, and little else. Fortunately, I always travel with plenty of cortisone and Benadryl; a quick trip to my carry-on bag, and the patient was cured.

That was over thirty years ago. I would hope that Alitalia has managed to modernize their medical kits since then, but one never knows.

• • •

I like to think of this somewhat surprising encounter as reflective of the Italians' casual approach to many things that we in the United States would handle with a touch more gravity or formality. For many, this is what is so attractive about Italian culture—life is lived with a certain joyful gusto that clings to tradition without being overly rigid, all the while maintaining a level of grace and dignity. There is even an undeniable element of charm in the ways they can prick the ego of the individual too self-important to get with their program. Life in Italy, while giving me a welcome view of old world pomp, also allowed me a somewhat bracing take on the ideas of social importance and self-importance, and certainly on the relative importance of the self-important physician.

As a first-year medical student in Rome, because I was an American, and as the result of basic differences in the Italian and American education systems, I was actually entered into the third year of a seven-year program. And, as if to add even more swagger to my step, all my neighbors would constantly address me as *dottore*. It was as if I was so far ahead of the game already that my neighbors in that ancient neighborhood could see me naturally wearing the mantle that I was then working to assume.

I will simply take it for granted that you, the reader, will be able to empathize with my chagrin when I found from some Italian fellow students that everyone who enters university, be it for accounting, education, or medicine, comes out with a doctorate degree, hence every university student is referred to as *dottore*. Upon completion of the student's program of study, the graduate is presented with a *laurea*, literally a "laurel," but in reality an olive branch , placed upon his or her head (compare this with our bachelor's degree, or *baccalaureate*, literally "half a laurel"). Despite my relative disappointment at the overall situation, it was hard not to be impressed with that magnificently Roman tradition that was still observed over fifteen hundred years after the fall of the empire.

I eventually learned that Italians love acquiring numerous titles throughout life, with each one finding its way onto their business or calling cards. It is not difficult to find someone who is not only a *dottore*, but also a *commendatore* (another kind of knight in the Italian system), a *professore* ... and the list goes on. Equal parts cultural pomp and societal ego-stroking, this phenomenon contributes to a certain surreal quality that many Americans find in European societies, but which seems especially resonant in Italy, the only culture in the world that could have produced both Mussolini and Fellini. But one night a few years ago, as I was sitting in a famous Roman restaurant called Sabatini's, an event occurred that was so strange Fellini himself couldn't have conjured it up.

As I sat in the dining room with my party, I became aware of an elderly couple, accompanied by another elderly man, at a table across the room. At some point during their spaghetti course, the male of the couple pitched forward face-first into his plate as if he had suddenly lost consciousness. Soon the other gentleman laid him out on the floor, where he took the stricken man's legs in his hands while standing over him, and began to sway them back and forth as if they were cross-country ski poles. After a few minutes everything seemed back to normal and they all resumed eating.

As bizarre as the scene appeared to me, I realized that no one else in the place seemed to pay any attention at all to the event. There were no cries of shock or alarm, no one rushed to the sick man's aid, no representative of management hovered worriedly nearby. It caused less stir than someone dropping a fork.

About a half-hour later, now in the middle of their main course, the scene repeated itself as the same man appeared to first go limp, then was placed upon the floor by his friend, who re-administered the original treatment. As everything again played out as it had earlier, a peddler managed to enter the restaurant carrying an armful of paintings, which he then diligently tried to hawk to the patrons. As he went table to table with his wares, everyone's attention was on the paintings while the old man on the floor with his legs in the air and food smeared across his face went unacknowledged. Again. This time, the man pumped his supine friend's legs for an exceptionally long time before the poor man began to come around. Unable to sit idly by at this point, I was compelled to go over and help these people. I crossed the room to the spot where these two men were engaged in this curious exercise, in front of the table where they were all dining moments before, and plainly stated with obvious concern, "I am a doctor from America, can I help?" Completely unperturbed, the woman of the party responded, "We don't need a doctor, we have Professor so-and-so." By now equal parts shocked and chastened, I returned to my dinner. Within moments, the "patient" got up and resumed his place at the table.

• • •

These experiences and others like them came at just the right time in my life and professional development. I have encountered more than one fellow doctor in my career to date who has somehow come to the conclusion that his or her particular level of social, financial, and professional accomplishment incurs the right to deal with others, such as patients, students and colleagues, as if from a pedestal of merit and hot air. The stories I've recounted here will always remind me that life offers us no shortage of ways to be humbled, and that each instance should be taken as a sign that no matter how important we think we are, there will always be something that takes us down a peg.

Not incidentally, this is how I also learned that sometimes long-lasting popular ideas can trump what we consider to be science and common sense. Besides being humbling, it was instructive in that it taught me that what passes for medicine in one culture might seem to approach witchcraft or a slapstick routine by the standards of another. I would eventually learn that not only can this perception cut both ways across a cultural divide, but it can be further aggravated by whatever the prevailing geopolitical rifts happen to be.

When I visited China in 1980 as part of a small group tour, one of our number suffered a heart attack as we toured the city of Shanghai. I volunteered to accompany the woman to the hospital, as I felt sure that receiving emergency cardiac care in a Chinese hospital at the height of the Cold War would be an intimidating prospect for an American tourist, and thought she would benefit from me being on-hand. Of course, I will also admit to a certain curiosity about the state of medicine in the People's Republic of China, a country our government seemed to deem a lesser threat than the U.S.S.R. but against whose army we had fought during the Korean War twenty-seven years earlier. So imagine my surprise when the ambulance that arrived to take us to the hospital was the very same type of crackerbox ambulance I had driven as a corpsman back in 1957. Once we were loaded in, I realized that the vehicle was most likely of World War II-vintage. And I soon got a good look at the conventional medical technology of the mighty Chinese nation: the doctor on duty with the ambulance crew was administering oxygen to the patient by means of a tire inner tube attached to a small catheter. As he squeezed the inner tube, air was propelled through the catheter and into the patient's lungs.

When we arrived at Shanghai's Sun Yat Sen Hospital, the woman was immediately checked in and was given an unexpected choice to make: she was offered the option of receiving treatment in the Western model or in the more traditional methods of Chinese medicine. Certainly overwhelmed by the fact that she was suffering a heart attack on the other side of the globe from everyone she knew and loved, the woman went with what she knew and without hesitation opted for Western treatment. In response, she was simply told to go to the third floor; no orderlies, nurses, or doctors stepped forward to assist or even accompany her. Already shocked, we soon realized that there were no elevators and that she was expected to walk to the third floor. I half expected the attending physician to ask the woman if she wouldn't mind being a dear and carrying his stack of charts, since she was going that way. I was growing increasingly impatient with the situation, and I put the woman in a chair and carried her up the stairs to the third floor with the help of our government tour guide who had accompanied us to the hospital. As the situation unfolded, I began to wonder if our treatment wasn't something of a silent rebuke for refusing treatment in the Chinese fashion. But I handed my fellow tourist over to the care of the hospital's staff and was assured that she would receive the proper care.

The following day our group left China for Hong Kong, which was then still a British colony. The group was having a farewell dinner to celebrate our last night in the People's Republic, when our tour guide was suddenly summoned to the hotel lobby. There he found our heart attack patient from the previous day. It seems that she had been released from the hospital only hours after being checked in and was transported to the hotel to rejoin the group before we crossed the border. Evidently the Chinese had a rule that if a certain number of people enter the country on a visa, that same number of people must depart on the same visa, heart attack or no.

I still can't help but wonder if she would have been treated differently had she opted for Chinese medicine over Western. Then again, perhaps she would have been discharged even faster if she had chosen traditional medicine.

• • •

A lesson to learn here is that, though you may expect certain standards and norms should you have a health alarm in a foreign country or when traveling anywhere away from home, you probably shouldn't. Be careful where you get sick—if you know you have a pre-existing condition, plan ahead. Or even postpone your trip. I'd much rather skip a vacation than risk being treated in a facility with a mindset that is a century or more out of date with modern science.

I realize that sounds harsh. Perhaps that quip was the result of cultural and/or professional bias that is by no means peculiar to Western medicine. We nearly all tend to feel that our social, professional, national, or ethnic group possesses a fundamental truth or level of "correctness" that other groups, due to their fundamentally benighted nature, just can't seem to pick up on. This particularly applies to the periodic face-offs between modern (as in "contemporary," and not necessarily meant as a value comparison) and traditional cultures, and even I can be guilty of such behavior from time to time.

So in an effort to soothe troubled brows, allow me to take this opportunity to explicitly acknowledge the following facts: it is eminently possible to receive proper, adequate, modern medical treatment nearly anywhere in the civilized world; old world geography does not necessarily mean old world medicine; and there are many millions of people worldwide who use what we would call "alternative medicine," in the form of traditional Chinese methods, the ancient Indian discipline called Ayurveda, or simple folk remedies that have managed to be passed along for generations.

I am addressing these three ideas here because there is a peculiar sense of overlap when people talk about one of these topics. The idea of getting sick while in a foreign land often fills the head with images of primitive treatment in questionable facilities, but some of these primitive treatments were preserved and sworn by on the parts of our parents and grandparents because they represented some concrete course of action against the previously mysterious specter of illness in an age before generally accessible healthcare.

According to a 2004 study by the National Institutes of Health, approximately 50% of Americans have used some form of "alternative therapy" at least once. And make no mistake that this designation includes many of the venerated folk remedies that tie us to the various ethnic and national heritages from which our forbearers came. Perhaps that is why some of us are so attached to them. After all, it's kind of difficult to completely and utterly reject a remedy that has close association with mom or grandma ministering to your needs as a child too sick to go to school, conjuring up feelings of safety and security as well as images of a beloved family member who may have long ago passed away.

With this in mind, there is specific reason that I chose to reference the image of a kindly grandmother in my heartwarming recollection of childhood illness. In Yiddish, the term for an old wives' tale is *bubbe mayse,* literally "grandmother's story." The term is particularly evocative in this case because it is these "moms with extra frosting," as one anonymously sentimental wit once described them, that are most often the conduits for the folk remedies—as well as some plainly incorrect ideas about health and illness—to which so many of us so stubbornly cling. If such ideas were good enough for nana, many of us say to ourselves, then it'll be good enough for me.

Well, just because mee-maw believed in it doesn't necessarily make it true. Some of the cures and ideas about health maintenance we cling to are simply wrong, some actually working against us rather than helping us stay healthy. For example, the idea that cotton swabs are safe and ideal for cleaning out your ears. In fact, one of the worst things you can do is stick anything into your ear canal and root around. All you do is push wax deeper into your ear while running the risk of puncturing the delicate membrane of your ear drum. Best to follow the advice given by Chesebrough–Ponds, the former maker of Q-tip-brand swabs, in an old advertisement for that product: never, ever stick anything in your ear besides your elbow.

More serious are the well-meaning fallacies that actively contribute to worsening a given illness or situation by persuading the sufferer that the condition being experienced is either much less serious or much more treatable than it actually is, or—even worse—that the conventional treatment is potentially more harmful than beneficial because it defies traditional folk knowledge. One example of this, a situation that bedevils healthcare professionals by the thousands every year, is the belief that one can contract influenza by receiving the flu inoculation. The flu vaccine, like any other, contains dead samples of its particular virus rather than the dangerous live one. The body may well develop some sort of reaction to the introduction of the dead virus sample into the system, but this is most certainly not how influenza is spread. Unfortunately the prevalence of this attitude, particularly among the elderly and recent immigrants from the developing world, puts untold numbers of potentially high-risk patients in danger of contracting a strain of influenza that could end up as more than just another case of the winter "icks." Of more recent vintage is the belief that taking acidophilus orally can treat or prevent a vaginal yeast infection. In reality, taking it orally would spread it through the body via its absorption in the digestive tract rather than concentrate it at the site of the infection, where it would do the most good.

There is yet another subset of long-standing myths that are so "out there" that I honestly can't understand how anyone could possibly believe them to be effective. Did you know, for instance, that there are some people who think that nailing a potato to a tree or spilling loose tea leaves from your teacup into a saucer will somehow soothe a toothache? One would assume that this "remedy" would be less effective in treating a headache brought on by hunger. Better that you eat the potato and drink the tea; at least you'll get a snack out of it. And if you find yourself with a headache or toothache of unusual intensity or duration, a visit to your doctor will do more to ease your pain than any amount of hammering.

All of that said, there are a number of old world, old-time remedies and pronouncements that are perfectly valid and effective. So rather than leave grandma with a blackened reputation as the result of my withering expose of pseudo-medical fallacies, I can immediately cite

Old World Remedies Versus New World Remedies

INEFFECTIVE "OLD WORLD" REMEDIES AND MYTHS THAT ARE NOT TRUE:

- *Going outside with wet hair or being in a draft will cause a cold.* False. Catching the bug that causes the cold is what does it.
- *Washing your hands will prevent catching a cold.* False. Colds are caught by inhaling droplets of microscopic cold virus coughed up by an infected person.
- *Crossing your eyes will make them get stuck in that position.* False. Although it might alienate some of your co-workers.
- *You can catch poison ivy by touching someone else's poison ivy rash.* False. You have to be allergic to poison ivy, not someone's rash.
- *You can get influenza from the flu shot.* False. The shot is made from dead virus samples and not the live toxic one.
- *Knuckle cracking causes arthritis.* False. This has yet to be proven.
- *You should wait one hour after eating before going swimming.* False. As long as there aren't ten-foot waves, swim away.
- *Shaving your hair will make it grow in coarser, darker, and faster.* False. If this were true, every balding man would be shaving his head.
- *We only use 10% of our brain.* False. We actually use 100% of it during the course of the day, although not necessarily all at once.
- *Nailing a potato on to a tree or spilling your tea leaves into a saucer, will make your headache go away.* False. Eat the potato and drink the tea. You may still have a headache, but at least you'll get a good meal out of it!
- *Kissing a baby's forehead will help you tell whether the child has a fever.* False. We can't say goodbye to the thermometer just yet.
- *By looking at someone's sore throat, we'll be able to tell if it's a strep throat.* False. You must take a culture to determine this.
- *Cotton swabs are a great way to clean your ear.* False. They actually push the wax deeper into the ear canal. Still, I wish I owned the company that makes Q-tips; they sure sell a lot for the wrong reason.
- *Holding a hot water bag or bottle to your liver will cure your liver ail-*

ment. False. Try taking an antacid or newer stomach medicine to treat the real problem: indigestion.

- *Taking acidophilus by mouth will prevent vaginal yeast infections.* False. See below.

"Old World" Prescriptions That Really Work

- Chicken soup does help in treating a cold. There are mucus-dissolving chemicals in chicken soup which help break up and drain a cold's congestion.
- If you don't have a thermometer, remember that a fever goes hand-in-hand with an increased heart rate, and that every extra ten points of one's pulse equals a one-degree rise in ones' body temperature, just like I told Gregory Hines all those years (and pages) ago.
- If you're having trouble sleeping, warm milk will help induce sleep because of the chemical tryptophan.
- If you're flying, two squirts of the nasal spray Afrin one hour before landing will usually prevent your ears from popping or your sinuses from hurting if you have a cold.
- Use of the strong underarm antiperspirant Mitchum on your feet every morning will help prevent your feet from perspiring and developing athlete's foot.
- Painting the inside of your metal jewelry (rings, earrings, etc) with clear nail polish will prevent allergic skin reactions to that particular piece.
- If you contract traveler's diarrhea and can't find Gatorade, do as they do in Rome—take a large glass of freshly squeezed lemon juice and add two teaspoons of salt and a tablespoon of sugar. It works just the same.
- To prevent vaginal fungus infections during a treatment with antibiotics, place plain, unflavored yoghurt in a piece of tinfoil, shape it in the form of a bullet, and freeze. Use as a daily vaginal suppository and you won't get the fungus (remove the tin foil first).
- Recurrent *Staphyllococcal* skin infections (including MRSA) and boils can actually be washed away by showering with "pHisoHex" soap twice a day for one month, but you'll need a prescription first.

> • If you need to know how much weight you have gained or lost, look at your belt buckle. The "Klein Observation Method" has proven that each notch on your belt, up or down, represents five pounds. Surprise your friends or family by checking out their belts and telling how much weight they lost or gained (perhaps not the latter).

two instances where she was right on the money. Chicken soup does, in fact, aid in the management of the common cold because the rendered fat and cooked-down vegetable extracts in the broth deliver chemicals that help the body break up and eliminate excess mucous (matzo balls optional). And if you are having trouble dozing off, it is true that warm milk will help induce sleep because it contains the essential amino acid tryptophan, the same chemical that makes falling asleep in front of the television on Thanksgiving a hallowed American tradition. But no milk if you have a cold; the notion of milk creating phlegm is false, but it does make the existing mucous thicker and harder to expel. And besides ... milk and chicken soup? Ewwww.

• • •

Of course, this still leaves us with the issue of healthcare quality in foreign lands and the problems of staying healthy while traveling. Just because your great-grandmother from Bialystok was in the habit of treating a chest cold with a poultice of chicken fat and horseradish does not mean that you should expect similar treatment if you fall ill while traveling in modern Poland. Still, being able to maintain your good health while traveling in a foreign land is no small concern. As my health-related travelogues from a few pages back demonstrate, illness or injury while traveling abroad can give a person intimidating choices to face in both an environment and a healthcare system that are utterly unfamiliar and therefore themselves intimidating. This has become an even more serious concern as Americans have become much more travel-savvy in the last thirty or so years, the growing global economy leading some of us to jobs in far flung cities like London, Riyadh, or Tokyo, and a fluctuating dollar driving more American retirees to places like Mexico, Portugal, and Costa Rica, where their savings will go further than it would here.

There is certainly an upside to this. As borders and cultural obstacles are leveled through travel and cooperation, knowledge and experience are shared across cultures that were once viewed as radically divergent. This new global vision gives the average individual greater leeway to learn about different social customs, business practices, and if lucky, courtship rituals. And of course the medical approaches and health perspectives of the dominant group in whatever region a person might find himself.

It should therefore be comforting to know that certain maladies that travelers experience are both quite common and fairly minor. Most of us are familiar with the terms "Montezuma's revenge" or "Roman tummy." Despite their exotically specific names, they are just different terms for a common ailment—traveler's diarrhea (usually shortened to just plain "diarrhea"). This most familiar of tourist afflictions, usually accompanied by abdominal cramps and a marked loss of appetite, is usually the result of either poor water sanitation— still common in developing countries—or the presence of microscopic organisms with which our bodies have no experience.[3] Nearly everyone who has traveled outside the United States has had a bout of the "travelin' trots." I had my own some years ago in east Jerusalem while on a family vacation, before Israel extended its public works system to that part of the newly re-unified city. When I learned that my sister-in-law was suffering from the same symptoms, I waited an extra two weeks before diagnosing her with a *Ghardia lamblia* infestation because she was losing weight she desperately needed to shed.

Usually it is quite easy to avoid serious problems, should you fall ill while traveling. All it really takes is a little preparation and forethought,

---

Travel Maladies and How to Handle Them

SIGNS & SYMPTOMS OF COMMON CONDITIONS FROM FOREIGN SHORES:
- Montezuma's revenge, Roman tummy, or traveler's diarrhea usually occur after one week, when most travelers are returning from vacation.

---

[3] Lest you think that such organisms are solely the province of developing countries, I remind you of the discovery of small harmless copepods (crusteceans) in the New York City water supply in the spring of 2004.

- Diarrhea, abdominal cramps, and loss of appetite may occur weeks after visiting cities with poor water sanitation and ski resorts.[4]
- Numbness and sometimes temporary paralysis can occur after eating certain coral reef fish in the Caribbean known to cause ciguatera, a foodborne illness caused by the accumulation of a naturally-occurring toxin in the bodies of these fish.
- A persistent cough developing 4 to 5 days after visiting certain cities or areas, such as Peking (due to dust) and the San Joaquin Valley (due to a fungus).
- Bloody urine may result after swimming in fresh water lakes in countries with poorly maintained agricultural areas which lack proper sanitation, such as Egypt, Japan and Puerto Rico; this is due to a parasitic infection resulting from fertilizer or other agricultural products or by-products leeching into the nearby bodies of water.
- Certain areas of South America have parasite-infected horse flies, the bites of which are the cause of their most common form of heart disease.

PRESCRIPTION

- For assistance both before and after falling ill, try the CDC website, call local health departments, experienced travel agents, or travel physicians.
- Vaccines against most diseases have to be started 1-2 months before your trip. Usual shots include: hepatitis A, tetanus toxoid, typhoid (the shot is more effective than the pill form); certain countries may require yellow fever vaccine, as well as one for cholera.
- Extended stays in poorer countries may necessitate vaccination against hepatitis B (given in three separate shots, months apart).
- Visitors to China, Japan, and other countries in the Far East may require the encephalitis vaccine.
- Travelers to malaria-plagued countries should start their preventive medications weeks before departure. Failure to do so will raise the risk of contracting this serious illness.

---

4 Because of extremely basic and often aftermarket plumbing at many ski resorts, sewage has been known to taint the drinking water lines.

- Upon return, one should get stool studies routinely if your itinerary included visits to Third World countries, ski resorts, or cities known for poor water sanitation; certainly, stool studies must be obtained if one has abdominal complaints.
- Bring with you all medicines that you regularly take, as there is no guarantee that they will be available where you are traveling.
- Travelers going to very high elevations (Peru, Colorado, etc.) may need a specific pill to combat altitude sickness.
- Contrary to popular belief, gastrointestinal infections are not best treated with antibiotics, as this increases the likelihood of entering the carrier state and may also lead to resistant bacteria. As a stop-gap measure, consume large amounts of Gatorade or a similar type of drink
- *Saccharomyces boulardii,* a probiotic yeast found in some tropical fruits and available in pill form, will prevent traveler's diarrhea and diarrhea caused by antibiotic treatment; simply take one tablet per day while traveling or on antibiotics.
- Acyclovir tablets can prevent sun blisters (fever sores) if taken hours before exposure, and are especially recommended for travel to the South.
- If you get sick while abroad, you may have brought an American disease with you. Keep this thought in the front of your mind, as we too have many diseases that are not common on foreign shores.
- Where appropriate, insect repellents and netting should be routinely used.
- Drink bottled water. If most Europeans drink it, they probably don't trust their own water either.

and a liberal dose of common sense. Since the most common health complaints for the traveler are the results of water borne organisms, relying on bottled water is one simple step to take, especially in areas with a reputation for such problems like Mexico, St. Petersburg in Russia, and the Sinai Peninsula in Egypt. I would even go so far as to advise you to pay attention to the condition of the bottle of water you buy, especially if purchased from a street vendor or in a particularly impoverished district. I have heard more than one tale of unscrupulous vendors filling empty spring water bottles with local tap water and selling them to unsuspecting tourists, with predictable results. It sounds funny until it happens to you.

Beyond that, use resources like the Center for Disease Control's website to research which illnesses are common to your destination well before departure, and which inoculations—if any—are indicated. Check with the local U.S. consulate to see whom they would recommend if a problem does arise. If you have life-threatening allergies or a pre-existing chronic condition, check ahead for an appropriately trained specialist and be sure to take any necessary medications with you, as they may not be available where you are traveling. In such a case, it might also be a good idea to have "emergency cards" printed up in the local language to inform a doctor or paramedic that you have a specific condition, an allergy to certain food ingredients or drugs, or that you require a specific treatment or remedy.

There are, however, always variables in any relatively complex equation (and here you thought you were done with algebra after the 10th grade). Sometimes our illness while abroad is the result of a "bug" unwittingly picked up while still at home. In some instances it may even be a condition unknown in your foreign destination. Lyme disease, for example, is only now becoming widely known outside North America. One of my patients was traveling in the south of France when she developed the classic bull's eye rash that indicates Lyme disease, which may appear two to three weeks after being bitten by an infected tick. This was some twenty years ago, and the seemingly unrelated list of symptoms combined with the mysterious rash had the French physicians flummoxed.

Language and other barriers aside, nearly all developed countries will have modern medical facilities that offer care and treatment on par with what you would expect to receive in Hometown, U.S.A. All you need to do is remember and act upon the old Boy Scout motto: Be Prepared.

Keeping the Faith

CULTURAL BARRIERS ARE IN NO WAY DEPENDENT on national borders in this day and age. (Indeed, were they ever?) Often enough, the source of misunderstanding is not the result of geographic location or opposing political systems, but the very beliefs that we hold and cherish as groups and individuals. How well do you know those in your neighborhood or community who are Hindu, Jewish, Muslim, or of other backgrounds that are numerical minorities in the Western world?

As a Jewish person, I am particularly aware of the misconceptions and mistrust that swirl around issues of religion and faith. And I am constantly amazed and dismayed at the irony of it all, how something that can be so inspiring and uplifting for some can manifest itself as something so rancorous and exclusionist in the minds and actions of others. I have always seen faith, the Jewish faith and others, as a great guide and motivator, a potential reflection of what is right with both people and the universe, and I would like to think that I have done my best to reach out to like minded people across the thresholds of our respective beliefs. That was how I developed and maintained my friendship with the Armenian Bishop of Jerusalem for so many years, a relationship of which I am immensely proud and for which I am deeply thankful. It's also how I helped start a friendship that would eventually lead me to not just one, but two experiences with Pope John Paul II.

Years ago, an Italian-speaking couple came into my office for a check-up, hearing that I was a physician who spoke Italian. The Fischettis had come from Rome after IBM transferred the husband, Massimo, to a research lab in the New York area. Though they each spoke English quite well, the Fischettis were glad to have a physician at their disposal with whom they could communicate in their native tongue, and I was equally glad to have new friends with whom to reminisce about Rome. One day Alessandra Fischetti brought in her mother, Elena, who had come to visit from Rome. It seems Elena suffered from severe, chronic allergies and needed regular shots to control her condition. When Alessandra asked me to administer the shots to her mother I saw no problem, provided Elena either had vials of her vaccine or had her physician's recommendation of a proper substitute if her normal vaccine was not available in the United States. As it turned out, she not only had the proper vaccine, but had brought the vial with her to the office. I sat Elena down and began to prepare her shot, but while checking the vials of vaccine I noted that her name was nowhere on the vial, which instead carried a man's name preceded by the title "Monsignor."

Realizing that she had received the wrong vaccine, she borrowed my telephone and called her husband, Mario, back in Rome. Mario Bresciani happened to be the highest lay employee in the office of the Secretariat of State of the Holy See, the Vatican's counterpart to our State Department. When Elena and Alessandra explained the situation to him, he insisted that I be put on the line. He thanked me and said that he would make sure that the correct vaccine would arrive in New York with the next day's diplomatic pouch. Sure enough, Elena came in the next day with the correct vaccine.

This scenario signaled the start of a long friendship with Mario and Elena, the parents in Rome. We kept in touch beyond Alessandra and Massimo's posting in New York, and I regularly visited them during my return trips to Italy. Mario, the gracious Roman host, was able to give me wonderful tours of Vatican City and its facilities and attractions, as well as grant me access to sights and events that most people only read about in the newspaper.

It was during one of these visits to Rome and Vatican City in 1994 that I received from Mario an invitation to a concert at the Vatican. But this was no ordinary musical performance. That year, Pope John Paul II had just established, for the first time in history, diplomatic relations between the Holy See and the State of Israel. To mark this momentous event, His Holiness helped to conceive and hosted The Papal Concert to Commemorate the Holocaust, a program of compositions by Beethoven and Leonard Bernstein mixed with Jewish liturgical music, all played by the Royal Philharmonic Orchestra and conducted by American maestro Gilbert Levine, and to which were invited the President of Italy, the Chief Rabbi of Rome, and cardinals from around the world. As an added gesture to this already stirring motion, the leader of the world's Roman Catholics invited 200 Holocaust survivors as his special guests.

In this noble company I was seated two rows in front of the Holy Father, with the seat next to me bearing a card that denoted it as reserved for an evidently high-ranking cardinal. As I sat waiting for the processional of the Pope and his cardinals to enter and the concert to then begin, a French gentleman sitting two seats away leaned over to get my attention. "Would you," he asked, "kindly take a picture of myself and my cousin, the Cardinal of Paris, who will be sitting next to you?" I agreed and he promptly handed me his camera. "My name is Seymour Weiss," he said as he shook my hand.

I introduced myself in turn and could not resist commenting on what I perceived as the incongruity of Mr. Weiss' seemingly Jewish name with the fact that he was related to the Catholic Cardinal of Paris. He responded that he was indeed Jewish, and that his cousin was also born Jewish, the son of Polish émigrés to France during the anti-Semitic upheavals that seemed to mark the independence movements of Eastern Europe after the First World War. Though his grandfather was a rabbi in Poland, young Aaron Lustiger was raised in a secular and enlightened household. During his early teens he began to read the New Testament and ended up deeply moved by it, converting to Catholicism at age 14. Though religious conversion is a landmark event in any person's life, it carried even more weight in Aaron's case. He turned 14 in the year 1940, one year after Germany initiated World War II, and converted on Good Friday of that year, a day known for centuries to European Jews as a time of pogroms by their Christian neighbors. It was only three months before the fall of Paris to the Nazis in June of 1940.

Though Aaron gained protection by posing as a seminary student when the Nazis began deportations of Parisian Jews in 1942, his mother had no such protection and was betrayed by one of her employees in the family shop. She was deported to Auschwitz, where she died the following year. But Aaron, now baptized as Jean-Marie, managed to escape with his father and sister to Orleans, where they lived in hiding until the end of the war. As he lived in hiding with his family, his Catholic faith grew and was strengthened, leading him to pursue ordination as a priest in 1954. As he rose steadily through the ranks of the Church, first as a chaplain at the Sorbonne, then through various academic and high-profile parish postings until becoming Bishop of Orleans in 1979, Archbishop of Paris in 1981, and Cardinal in 1983, he was driven by two imperatives. One was to bolster and communicate the beauty of his faith to those who had grown distant from the Church, as well as to ensure religious continuity for the next generation. The other was to bridge the gap between Christians, his brothers in faith, and Jews, the people of his blood and heritage. In one of his most famous quotes addressing both his Christian and Jewish detractors, each one believing him to be too much of one thing and too little of another, he said upon becoming archbishop: "I was born Jewish and so I remain, even if that is unacceptable for many."

His work and dedication caught the attention of the then new Pontiff, who was responsible for Lustiger's elevation to Bishop in 1979, and a warm friendship developed between the two men that lasted until their respective deaths. The two shared much in common: a Polish heritage, a deep love of the Church and her teachings, and hard yet lasting lessons from the tragedy of the Holocaust. Individually and together, these simple yet great men revived the traditions and stature of the Roman Catholic Church while doing everything in their respective powers to challenge and, as much as they could, eliminate an aspect and sensibility of Christianity that, while never an actual article of faith, was a grim constant in its dealings with the people that John Paul himself would publicly describe as Christians' "older brothers in faith" when he made his historic appearance at Rome's Great Synagogue in April of 1986.

Cardinal Lustiger soon made his entrance in procession with many cardinals from throughout the world. As he approached, I had to stand up to let him in my row and he pleasantly greeted me as he went to take his seat. However, upon seeing his long lost cousin sitting in the row behind us, he burst out with a broad smile.

• • •

Though he has only recently left us, John Paul II's program to improve the Church's relations with the Jewish People is already one of the most obvious legacies of his papacy. His desire to pursue this goal stemmed from his own experiences with Nazi occupation and oppression in his native Poland. His boyhood relationships with his Jewish neighbors in his hometown of Wadowice are well documented and were by all accounts close and cordial; his best friend was a Jewish boy named Jerzy Kluger, and the future Pope, then known by his birth name of Karol Wojtyla, was a regular player for the local Jewish youth soccer team. The dark years of 1939–45 showed him images that would haunt him for the rest of his life: neighbors being stripped of their land, their belongings, their dignity, and finally their lives, all as a matter of course at the hands of the German invaders. But perhaps more troubling to the devout young man were the silent acceptance and often active participation of his fellow Poles in the madness, degradation, and slaughter of those awful years, and the seeming refusal or inability of the Church to address the heinous crimes directed against their neighbors, fellow children of God. The rest of his life was dedicated, at least in part, to righting that titanic wrong that harmed Jew and Catholic alike. A result of his tireless work has been not only a better dialogue between Jews and Christians, but a renewed interest in religion as a unifying force rather than a dividing one, a way to further knowledge rather than stymie it, something that would bridge barriers rather than create them.

It was these beliefs of his that stood me in good stead during my second experience with the Pope. It was early in 1996, and His Holiness had just come off a year of activity that further stoked his reputation as a maverick reformer. He met with Nelson Mandela after his election to the South African presidency. He made the first ever Pastoral visits to Kenya and then-war-torn East Timor, and said Mass in each respective country's native tongue. He traveled to Manila for the tenth World Youth Day[5], where he celebrated Mass before a crowd of over five million, the largest-ever papal crowd, and widely believed to be the single largest Christian gathering in history. There he was targeted for assassination for the third time in his papacy, this time by a little known organization called al-Qaedea. And he made the unprecedented move of offering official apologies on behalf of the Church for the burnings-at-the-stake and religious wars that followed the Protestant Reformation, as well as the injustices committed against women in the Church's name.

Pope John Paul II's reputation is based not only on the greatness of his deeds, but upon the amazing and grueling pace he was able to maintain as leader of the world's one billion-plus Catholics. So I was

---

[5]   A celebration of the Roman Catholic faith geared toward the world's young people, conceived and initiated by Pope John Paul himself in 1984.

certainly impressed and excited when Mario told me that he was able to arrange for me to be present during one of John Paul II's more intimate audiences with members of the clergy and select faithful. The very idea of me, a Jewish guy from the Lower East Side of Manhattan, getting a chance to interact with His Holiness the Pope—let alone *this* pope, a figure so dynamic and compelling to the worlds of both politics and culture—was both terribly intimidating and completely irresistible.

Mario instructed me to meet him at the Bronze Door, an ornate and largely ceremonial portal to the Apostolic Palace, the residence of every pope since 1871. We met at the appointed time of 6:30 A.M., and I was then escorted into a tiny chapel next to the papal bedroom. In the chapel's rearmost pews sat some cardinals and Vatican clergy, but I was directed to a spot alongside two other Americans, a married couple, at the front of the room, where we sat only one chair's space away from the seat reserved for John Paul himself.

The Pope was in the habit of spending the first hour of his morning, 6:00–7:00, in silent prayer in his private quarters, and the small assemblage waited patiently for His Holiness to appear. At exactly 7:00 Pope John Paul II appeared in the chapel and celebrated the Mass with us for an hour. As he performed his sacred duties upon the room's beautiful altar, we three American visitors were directly behind him. The fact that we were in such close proximity to such a massive figure—one of the world's few remaining great monarchs, really—was awesome in itself. However, one could practically feel the energy and charisma emanating from his physical person. As much as being touched by his devotion and impressed by his station, one could feel the electricity of his personality. Though secure in and committed to my own Jewish heritage, it was impossible for me not to be deeply moved as I sat there.

I was suddenly jolted out of my reverie by the figure of a man jumping out from behind the altar. It turned out to be the official photographer, who immediately started shooting pictures of the Pope and his three guests. Just at that moment, His Holiness turned to me and appeared to offer me something. Though momentarily caught off balance both by the photographer and the fact that I was suddenly face to face with Pope John Paul II, I quickly realized that the Pope was in the middle of celebrating the sacrament of the Eucharist and was offering me a chance to partake of the host, the thin unleavened wafer that represents the body and the sacrifice of Jesus Christ.[6] It seems that I was standing in a spot that made me first in line to receive this sacrament.

Being Jewish, I had never found myself in this situation before. Now, not only was I receiving an invitation to participate in one of the holiest rituals of Christianity, administered by the hand of the spiritual leader of over one sixth of the world's population, but the entire scene was being immortalized on film by the Vatican photographer. If only I had been seated to the left of the couple, rather than the right! I certainly did not want to cause any sort of or problem or disruption during such a solemn and inspiring moment; so I accepted, meaning no disrespect whatsoever.

After the conclusion of the Mass, I was lucky enough to be able to speak with the Holy Father directly. I knew what a momentous and unique opportunity this was, and I made a conscious decision to make the most of it. Addressing him in Italian, and inasmuch as I was qualified to do so, I offered him a blessing for doing so much to extend the Church's hand to the Jewish people and put centuries of misunderstanding and enmity behind us. He thought about things for a moment or two and responded in English, "And I bless your family." I was struck by the fact that he did not mention my faux pas in taking communion, which is expressly forbidden to those not of the Catholic faith.

• • •

When I left my audience with the pope, I was escorted through the Apostolic Palace by the Pope's secretary, a Bishop whose name I do not recall. As he made conversation, asking me how I had enjoyed my meeting, I confessed my ignorance in accepting the Eucharist. When he heard my story, he just smiled and said, "You just had your first Holy Communion, and it was performed by His Holiness!"

When the Pope and I finally said good-bye, he handed me a beautifully ornate set of rosary beads. Each pope had his own special set of

---

6 According to Roman Catholic theology, when Jesus made the declaration, "This is my body," at the Last Supper, the very substance of the bread was converted to that of his body. The Church holds that the same transformation occurs at the consecration of the host and wine during the Eucharist ceremony, a doctrine known as *transubstantiation*.

rosary beads designed especially for him. Some popes give these as gifts, which are obviously blessed before being given to the recipient. The significance of such a gift and its value as an aid in prayer is immense, perhaps immeasurable. Even so, I had no use for them other than as a souvenir. So rather than keep them simply for the sake of having a memento, I felt that the proper thing to do was to give them to someone who could both enjoy them and benefit from using them.

I gave them to my friend Frank Yozzo, a devout Roman Catholic who had accompanied me to Rome for this trip, but whom I could not manage to bring with me to the unexpected papal audience. As it happened, Frank had the misfortune of having many members of his family afflicted with cancer and terminally ill. His brother Nicholas, a patient of mine, was especially far along, suffering from metastatic lung cancer. Not long before our departure for Vatican City, I had to inform him that given the advanced stage of his cancer, he had only six months to live. The scenario was particularly unpleasant for all of us. It is never easy to tell a patient the worst possible news a doctor can give, and it is even less pleasant to be the one receiving the dreadful news. On top of it all, both Nicholas and I were pained by Frank's suffering over the potential decimation of his family; he as a brother and I as a friend. With no other options available, Frank gave the Rosary beads to Nick and both hoped for a miracle.

Einstein once said: "Scientists were rated as great heretics by the Church, but they were truly religious men because of their faith in the orderliness of the universe." It may seem incongruous for a man of science to believe in miracles, but believe in them I do, as did Einstein. After receiving the blessed Rosary beads from Frank, Nick prayed the Rosary every day. Somehow, against the odds and the dictates of medical science, Nick went into remission and lived for another five years. Soon after his recovery, the brothers decided to give the beads to their sister who was also battling cancer. Miraculously (or so it seemed), she was able to beat cancer completely and lived for many more years.

• • •

Though science has outpaced religion for many as the discipline that provides the fundamental answers we all seek, the significance and impact of faith can be immense and, in some cases, life altering. And despite mankind's unfortunate history of discrimination, hatred, and violence in the name of this or that religious idea, the idea of religion itself can cut across any number of barriers to unite people—even those who may adhere to different philosophies—in the simple yet profound beauty of its basic concept: that there is an overarching power, called "God" by some and "The Greater Good" by others, which comes to our aid in times of need.

The key component to this idea is the notion of faith, a deep and driving belief in a greater figure or concept. What many people fail to grasp is that faith need not be exclusively of the religious variety, but can also be placed in a person, philosophy, or inanimate thing; it is simply a strong belief that exists beyond fully established or easily discernable fact.

There is a quote from George Bernard Shaw that seems especially apropos here. A well-lettered, pacifistic socialist-bordering-on-utopian idealist, he nonetheless had strongly held beliefs that would seem to contradict the greater theme of his personality and philosophy. One of these was his near complete rejection of medical advancements in surgery and vaccination, choosing to rely instead on judicious public sanitation, diligent personal hygiene, and a completely vegetarian diet. He famously expounded on some of these beliefs in his middle period play *The Doctor's Dilemma*, the premise of which is that physicians must balance their obligation to care for their patients with the need to perform what Shaw believed were unnecessary procedures (vaccination against smallpox, for instance, and seemingly any surgical procedure, regardless of the condition to be treated) in order to earn their livelihoods. His attitude in this respect was further encapsulated in one of his most famous quotes, of which there are many: "We have not lost faith, but we have transferred it from God to the medical profession."

Though I have already spent a fair number of pages pointing out a fair number of foibles of the medical everyman ("everydoctor"?), it's not a bad thing to have some measure of faith in the skills and knowledgeability of your doctor. As I have already said, there is nothing wrong with asking questions, offering opinions, or seeking a second medical opinion. But, while a doctor is just as human and fallible as any other person, that doesn't mean the doctor-patient relationship and information processes need to be contrarian or adversarial. After all, he or she did go to school for an awfully long time.

But while it is important to have such faith in your chosen healthcare professional, it is even more important to have some faith in the person you should know the best—yourself. Whether religious or atheist, thinker or doer, philosopher or follower, we all know (at least, we should) that our thoughts have the power to inspire and convince others and ourselves. From "Everything is possible for him who believes," in the Gospel of Mark, to the "if you believe it, you can achieve it" slogan found in so many self-help books and motivational posters, a belief and faith in one's self has long been an acknowledged component in the formula for success and achievement. This holds just as true when battling illness. If you have a fervent belief that you will recover, your chances of actual recovery can significantly increase.

To deconstruct the issue even further, faith is worthless—indeed, impossible—without a sense of meaning and purpose. This simple idea forms the basis, believe it or not, for an entire school of psychotherapy that itself further bears out the potential impacts of the ideas of faith and purpose. The school of thought is called logotherapy, from the ancient Greek *logos*, or "meaning," and is the brainchild of Viktor Frankl, one of the most eminent names in the history of psychology. Though he is generally cited alongside the names of his colleagues and contemporaries Sigmund Freud, Carl Jung, and Alfred Adler as a foundational figure, it is Frankl's logotherapy that relies most on the personal experiences of its founder. Viktor Frankl began his career in the mid 1920s in Vienna, then a veritable hotbed of the developing discipline of psychotherapy, and focused his work and research on the topics of depression and suicide. He was successful enough with his approaches to the two related problems that he was able to keep practicing as a physician, though with serious restrictions, until 1942, long after most Jews had been barred from the professions and imprisoned . But his abilities as a researcher and clinician were only able to protect him for so long, and in 1942 he and his family were finally deported from Vienna and given over to the modern barbarians of the Nazi S.S. and their system of extermination camps.

As he spent seemingly endless years, both before and after his deportation, witnessing the nearly unimaginable cruelty dished out by humans with essentially limitless power over other humans who had been stripped of even the most rudimentary powers and dignities of everyday life, he was able to more clearly formulate the doctrine he had developed before the war that had been so successful in dealing with even the most hopeless cases of depression and suicidal thought. The field that would come to be known as logotherapy posits that life always has meaning, even under the most miserable of circumstances, and that our motivation to survive and keep on living is our will, our inherent drive, to find meaning in life. It then follows that we have both the freedom and the instinct to find meaning in everything we do and experience, and in the actions (or inactions) we take when faced with suffering or sorrow that is beyond our ability to immediately change.

The relevance of this approach to Frankl's experience, the direct relation of one to the other, should require no further elucidation. But the lessons that can be learned by each and every one of us are immeasurable. Frankl's experience is demonstrable proof that we can each use our innate power to determine our own attitudes to any crisis, even serious illness, and choose a meaningful response to whatever life puts before us. The keys to doing so lie at the intersection where faith and meaning come together, and the ways they do so ... the ways we *make* them do so. When we believe that things happen for a reason, whether that reason seems to be divine or biological or circumstantial, we find meaning not only in our situation, but in our selves. This, in turn, can be a source of faith in our battles against seemingly insurmountable obstacles of nearly any sort, a most effective tool when the faith is placed in yourself and your own abilities/odds as much as in a higher power or purpose.

Of course, we all know that there are times when even the most "can-do" type of attitude will not be enough to win the fight. But even in those most desperate of situations, some level of positivity— fighting attitude, a refusal to give in to the darkness—can mark the difference between maintaining or losing a fundamental part of your dignity, your humanity, a part of your unique self that is perhaps indefinable. When she found out she had lung cancer, my first wife said: "If people can survive the horrors and the torture of concentration camps, I will survive this disease." Sadly, she did not survive. But she *did* exhibit the courage to fight back, and in so doing we lived three lifetimes during an emotional roller coaster that certainly handed us our fair share of disasters and disappointments but, along the way those last few months, also a surprising number of unexpected highs.

Since then, I have developed a deepened sense of respect and even inspiration from my work with patients who have had to overcome severe handicaps or endure fatal illnesses with their heads held high every step of the way, despite gloomy outlooks and often excruciating pain. I have cared for dying cancer patients, patients with the slow killer ALS (more commonly known as Lou Gehrig's disease), and other diseases that offered them no hope for survival, and watched them work through their plights with a level of dignity and grace that would perhaps leave the Dalai Lama speechless. I presently care for two wheelchair-bound patients with severe multiple sclerosis, and despite the fact that their bodies are literally wasted, they continue to smile even as they struggle to do the most basic of tasks. I don't know if I could do what they do, but they are the patients that really charge my emotional and professional batteries, and I make sure to tell them so. They are perhaps the most inspirational people I have ever personally encountered.

Don't ask what the meaning of life is; ask how you can give more meaning to your life. If you embrace the challenges in your life and flow with them rather than resist them, you will not only suffer less but, like the art of Tai Chi, you'll use the power of the seeming "foe" to transform the circumstance into a victory. In the end, even if your life (or that of a loved one) doesn't turn out as you hoped for, you will have lived a richer life than most.

Never underestimate the power of faith—any type of faith—when dealing with a medical situation, no matter how simple or grave.

The Holy Land Connection

T HOUGH I AM FASCINATED BY and possessed of a great respect for both the idea of faith and the truly good hearted faithful, there is something I should add: I myself am not a man of religious faith. Though I am proudly and unapologetically Jewish, my relation to the Jewish people is a relationship based on culture rather than religious observance. I bring this up here not simply because I've just spent the last several pages praising faith in general (religious and otherwise), but because of the unique place reserved for Jews and matters that relate or seem to relate directly to Jews in the equation of current events. Between the contemporary numerators of terrorism, liberation struggles, and refugees, and the denominators of security and a transparent, polyglot society, we Jews often find ourselves in unenviable positions.

This rings particularly true as many wags on the extreme left and right of the political spectrum attempt to use certain aspects of Jewish history against the *de facto* Jewish homeland, Israel, in an effort to define problems at home here in America as well as abroad. And while it is true that the unfortunate situation in the Middle East is inextricably bound up with the Israeli-Arab state of affairs, there is much that the public neither knows nor understands about the situation, despite the fact that Israel and her problems have been news nearly every day for the last forty years. As an intern at New York Medical College and again at later times in my career, I was able to visit Israel in some of her most trying hours and was able to see and learn things, in the social realm as well as the medical, that I feel the need to share in an effort to put a more practical and human face on a nation and a problem that so few fully and truly understand.

• • •

During my internship we had a three-month elective that could be spent in any major training center throughout the world. It was a chance to be exposed to a great professor or teaching program different than ours. The federal Department of Health's Department of Children's Welfare subdivision offered a program wherein a physician would volunteer to travel to Third World countries to evaluate programs that the department sponsored. The year was 1967, and the U.S. government was giving various grants to medical scientists in various countries who were engaged in projects geared toward improving health benefits for children. There was an interesting program in Yugoslavia which would have required me to travel from city to city to observe institution of these treatment programs throughout that country. It seemed like a worthy project, and Eastern Europe was at that time still shrouded in mystery for many Americans, so I applied and I was accepted.

Then, in the early summer of 1967, war broke out in Israel. Despite being Jewish, I had never had the urge to visit, study, or work in the renascent Jewish homeland. But the war seemed to turn on a switch, beckoning me to that place. So I changed my elective assignment from Yugoslavia to Israel, which was considered a Third World country in 1967 and did have a few qualifying research projects going on.

One project involved the study of fetal death and efforts to find the cause, and therefore the cure. It wasn't my field, but it seemed interesting. The project was being undertaken in Jerusalem; at the oldest OB-GYN Hospital in that city: Misgav Ladach, founded by the Sephardic[7] Jewish community in the 1850's. My job was to follow all diabetic and obese mothers until birth. It was in this subgroup of patients that the project director, Dr. Maccabi Salzberger, was interested, feeling that better control of these two entities would lower fetal wastage. Since that wouldn't occupy eight hours of work a day, my full time job was to include being on call, delivering babies that the attending midwives had difficulty with. Another function was to close episiotomies, which midwives were forbidden by law to do. I found this to be a scary proposition. Although I had delivered fifty babies as a medical student the year before, how could I be better equipped than these ladies who had delivered thousands? (Thankfully, everything worked out just fine.)

---

7   Sephardic Jews, or *Sephardim,* are Jews who trace their ancestry through Moorish Spain; perhaps the most famous of these was Moses Maimonides, who has left his mark on medicine to this day, and whose name is borne by numerous hospitals and educational institutions.

More intimidating, though, was the fact that due to Israel's reconquest of the entirety of Jerusalem we had to take over the duties of the Arab east Jerusalem OB-GYN hospital. There pre-natal care was non-existent, and women were continually brought in for immediate delivery without ever having seen an O.B. over the course of their pregnancies. It turned out to be a wonderful three-month learning experience, and I was able to befriend Arab and Israeli alike.

In fact, despite what the popular image may be outside Israel, there was a widespread sense of optimism immediately after the 1967 war among both the Israeli Jews and the former Jordanian Arabs that now found themselves on the other side of the border. Jerusalem in the summer of 1967 was a most interesting place. There seemed to be no outward hostility between Arabs and Jews, and life was marching on after the war. Arabs who hadn't seen their relatives or Jewish friends for twenty years were now allowed to come into Israel proper and look them up. Poor Arab women were taken in as housekeepers and young Arab men were given jobs in construction. As for the Jewish population, rather than being annihilated or pushed into the sea as their enemies had promised, the country was vibrant, exciting, safe, and secure. Jews were now allowed to visit and pray at the Western Wall (the wall that surrounded the famed Holy Temple and the holiest site in the world for Jews), and my colleagues and I were able to walk through the West Bank and eat at Arab restaurants without concern or fear.

One of the most fascinating figures to cross my path during this time was the director of my research project, Dr. Maccabi Salzberger. He was a handsome man, loved by the women of Jerusalem , both Jewish and Arab, and had a devoted following of patients from across the Middle East, including the wife of the Shah of Iran. His father had been a beloved physician to many Arab families before 1948, and though he had died during the twenty-year partition, well known Arabs came visiting Maccabi on an almost daily basis, many of them coming to Israel for secret therapy in direct violation of the laws of their respective countries. His wife, Lotte, was also something of a local celebrity. Descended from an old, wealthy German Jewish family, Lotte was one of the witnesses for the prosecution in the trial of war criminal Adolf Eichmann and would go on to be deputy mayor of the city of Jerusalem under the great Teddy Kollek. In 1967 she sat on the Jerusalem City Council and was also in charge of the School of Social Services at the Hebrew University. They both knew everybody in the Israeli political world, and repeated invitations to their weekly dinner parties put me in contact with Israel's great leaders: Yitzhak Rabin, Moshe Dayan, Ezer Weizman, and Golda Meir. The intellectual content and talk of the future was exciting and mind-boggling for me, a twenty-nine year old intern.

And for the first time in my life, I now spoke and understood Hebrew. The sense of connection I felt was immense as I spoke the ancient language while visiting archeological digs and watching farmers develop agriculture out of the desert. The sense of wonder was nearly overwhelming.

Still, there were a few instances in which the nearness of the hostilities was brought home. Every time Maccabi took us to dinner deep in Arab areas, or when some of his Arab patients, who were also long-time friends, invited us to Ramallah or some city not on the tourist list, Maccabi would always silently strap his pearl handled revolver to his side. While speaking to many Jewish and Arab families in Jerusalem, they would tell stories of bullets and bombs exploding near or even in their homes. Some friends showed us their apartments hit by ricochet bullets. The war was that close.

• • •

Though my experiences in Israel were overwhelmingly positive, I had no desire to return. That is until six years later, when Israel was attacked on all fronts on the holiest day of the Jewish calendar, Yom Kippur. As I sat in synagogue in Westchester with my family that day, word worked through the audience that there was a sneak attack on Israel similar to the Pearl Harbor attack thirty-two years earlier, catching the country unaware and jeopardizing the lives of all its citizens. I felt frustrated and helpless and wanted to be back, to help in any way I could. After one week of calling the Israel Embassy to no avail, I called my American colleagues Steve and Gerry who were studying in Israel.

I telephoned Gerry's wife, Nora, to learn his whereabouts, and Nora said she would get a message to him. It turned out that at the outbreak of hostilities they had hitched a ride into the desert with an army unit and volunteered as combat physicians, despite the fact that they were neither Israeli citizens nor members of the Israeli Defense Force. Four hours after my call to his wife, Gerry returned my phone call from a field phone in the Sinai Desert. "Yes, get on a plane to Israel and we'll work together."

Three days later I boarded an El Al jet at John F. Kennedy Airport, entrusting my family to the strong stewardship of my wife and my practice to colleagues. The flight was delayed for the boarding of Israel's Prime Minister Golda Meir, who was on her way back to Jerusalem from last-minute talks with President Nixon. She passed through the cabin and greeted all of us and then disappeared to the very front. I had these visions of her walking down the aisles later, serving chicken soup. But she was the serious leader of a country at war.

By the time we arrived in Israel, her negotiations with President Nixon had borne obvious fruit. Mrs. Meir had pressed the president for needed arms shipments, which were held up for whatever political motives Nixon had. However, as we deplaned at the airport outside of Tel Aviv we saw the giant Hercules C-130 transport planes circling overhead. They were sent from U.S. military bases in Europe and were filled with tanks, trucks, and artillery.

Friends picked me up and drove me to my first duty assignment. The Israeli Defense Force had converted a large sports stadium, Kfar Maccabi, into a prisoner-of-war camp for wounded Arab soldiers and pilots, and I was to be one of their medical doctors, caring for their wounds and infections and in charge of their IV hydration. The Israeli physicians tending to the enemy wounded were professional and treated the prisoners with the same care afforded to the Israeli wounded. Quite an unusual experience, considering some friend or colleague could have been killed by these same wounded prisoners, and quite in contrast to the tales of mistreatment brought back by returning Israeli prisoners (and, incidentally, confirmed by Arab "defectors" from Syria and dissidents from Lebanon). Still in all, I am sure the Israeli doctors were pleased that the American volunteers relieved them of caring for their enemies.

At that time, the entire country of Israel had only one infectious disease expert, Dr. Dan Michiele. At the start of the war he was appointed to lead the Israeli Defense Force's Medical Corps. Two days after my arrival, the word got out that I specialized in infectious diseases and phone calls began coming in from all the major treating hospitals, the most urgent from the burn center at the military hospital at Tel HaShomer, the central headquarters of the Israeli military establishment.

That war saw the extensive use of phosphorus missiles, which did their damage by generating extreme heat which enabled them to melt through tank armor. Tank crews on both sides were suffering high burn casualties, with their associated complications, including serious infections. Subsequently, another interesting problem arose: there appeared to be an excessive rate of rare superinfections with bacteria most had never heard of. So in the morning and afternoon I was assigned a medical translator who travelled with me from hospital to hospital to study the charts of the patients with rare infections. At night it was back to the burn center.

Perhaps because of their experiences with too many wars, Israel was able to reduce the time period involved in getting the wounded from front-line to rear permanent treating hospital to the quickest of any other army before, including the U.S. military. A wounded soldier was treated at the battlefield, then brought back to a field hospital, evacuated via helicopter, and finally brought to the treatment hospital. At every step of the way, each soldier was administered antibiotics, so that by the time he arrived at the hospital, he had received four varying sets of antibiotics. There were even twenty or thirty soldiers with kidney stones (due to the desert heat) who also received four sets of antibiotics, and one "shell shocked" soldier who also received the same treatment. The rule was to give antibiotics to all casualties.

What was happening was the various antibiotics were killing off all the susceptible organisms. The ones that weren't destroyed were normally in the body in minute amounts; but now that the massive amounts of susceptible bacteria were killed off, the rare ones flourished. The hospitals were fearful of cross contamination with these bacteria that one usually never hears of causing infections. The answer was simple: stop the multiple broad-spectrum antibiotics at each stage of evacuation. One only needs low dose penicillin or its equivalent in allowing patients to fight off the bacteria that could end up killing a wounded soldier within a day or two. Our recommendations were accepted and Dan Michiele incorporated our suggestions into the standard treatment manual of the I.D.F. Years later, my friend and colleague Steve Berger reported that he was told that the U.S. army had adopted the same treatment plan.

• • •

After the war, I was presented with a campaign medal and a letter of appreciation from the Israel government. For my care of the Egyptian wounded, the Egyptian government sponsored a wonderful tour in 1978, after the historic peace accord between Jerusalem and Cairo. During my tour, I met a former medical officer from the Egyptian army who helped care for Israeli prisoners during that same war. Interestingly, his name was Dr. Levi and he was then the leader of the tiny Egyptian Jewish community that remained after Nasser expelled most of the country's Jews in 1956. Ironically enough, we met in Cairo during Passover, when Jews around the world recall the Exodus from that land. I can still remember how we spent all night talking about our similar experiences, and can't help but think that there are innumerable and multi-layered lessons to learn not only from our individual experiences, but from taking the greater experience in its entirety. But rather than spell it out via my pronouncements, I will this one time leave it to you the reader to meditate on the unfortunate contradictions and repetitions that seem to characterize both that part of the world and, more and more, our own.

PHOTO ALBUM

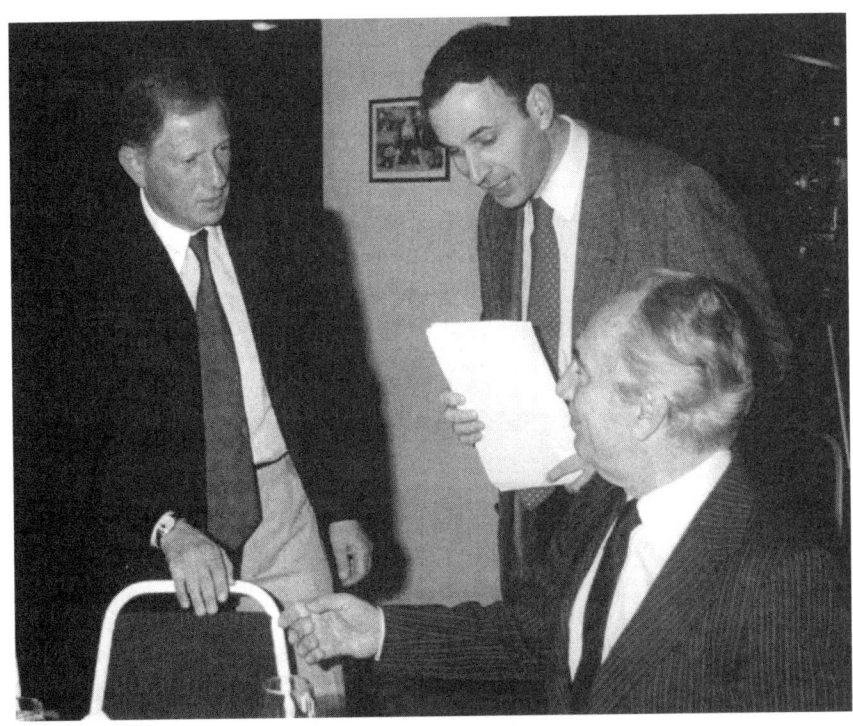

Meeting with former Israeli Prime Minister Shimon Peres

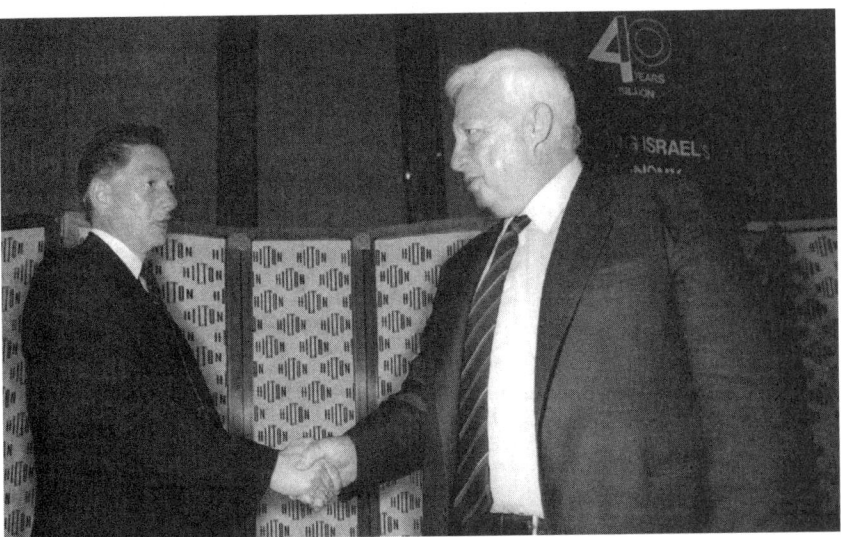

Shaking hands with another former Israeli Prime Ministrer, Ariel Sharon, at a state dinner in Jerusalem

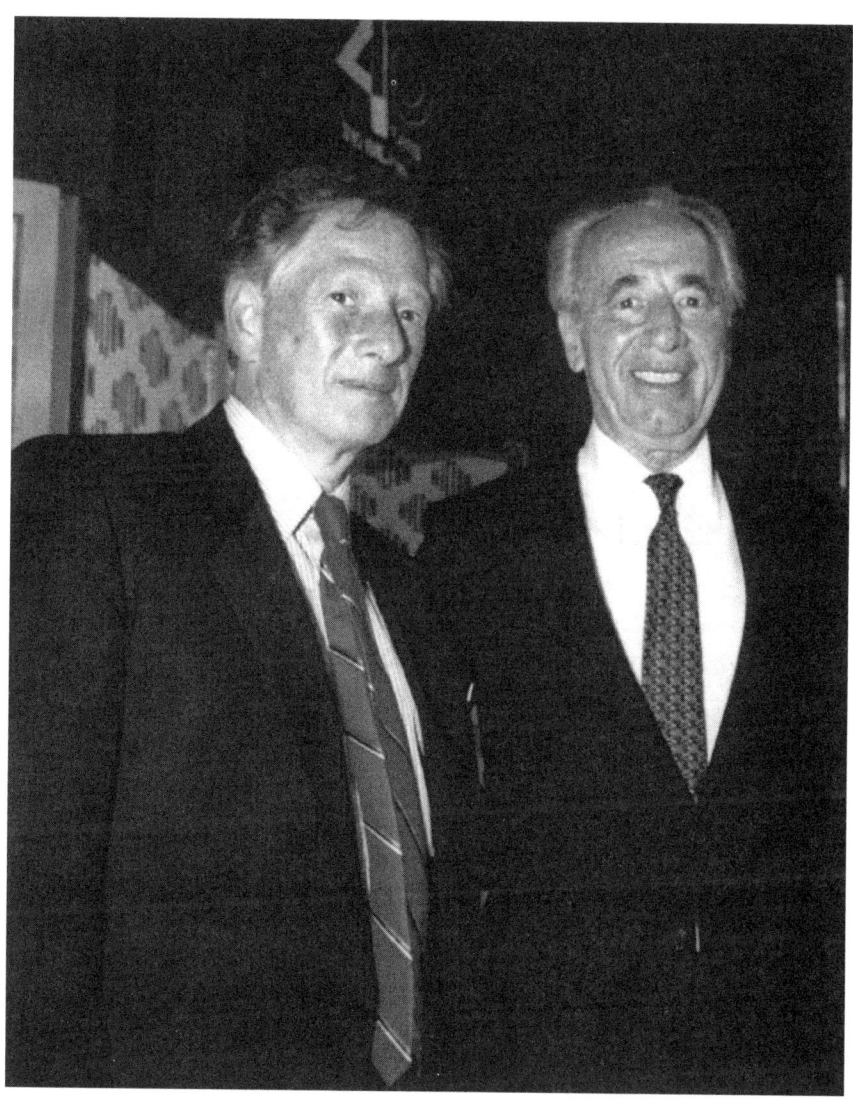

With diplomat Shimon Peres in Tel Aviv

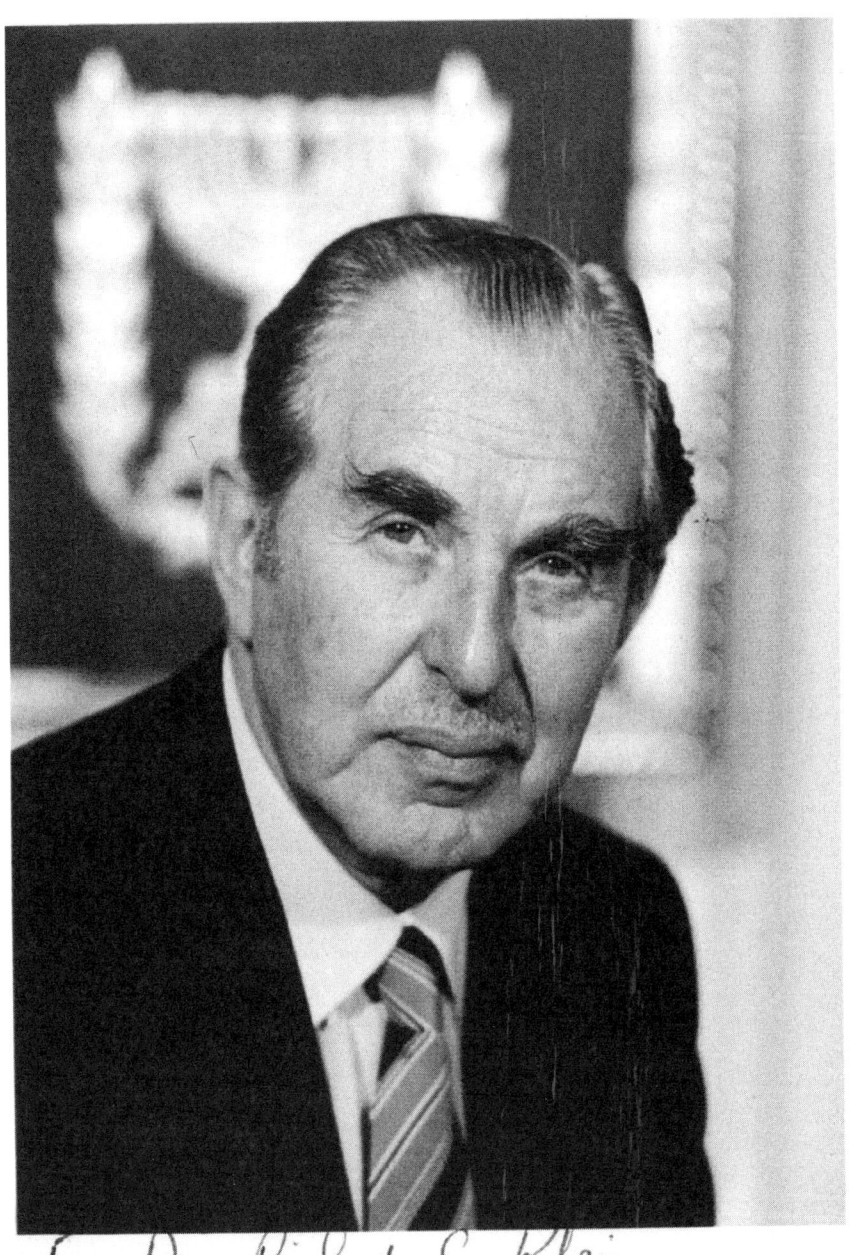

For Dr. Richard S. Klein
On your 50th birthday.
Chaim Herzog. 20 Nov.
1988.

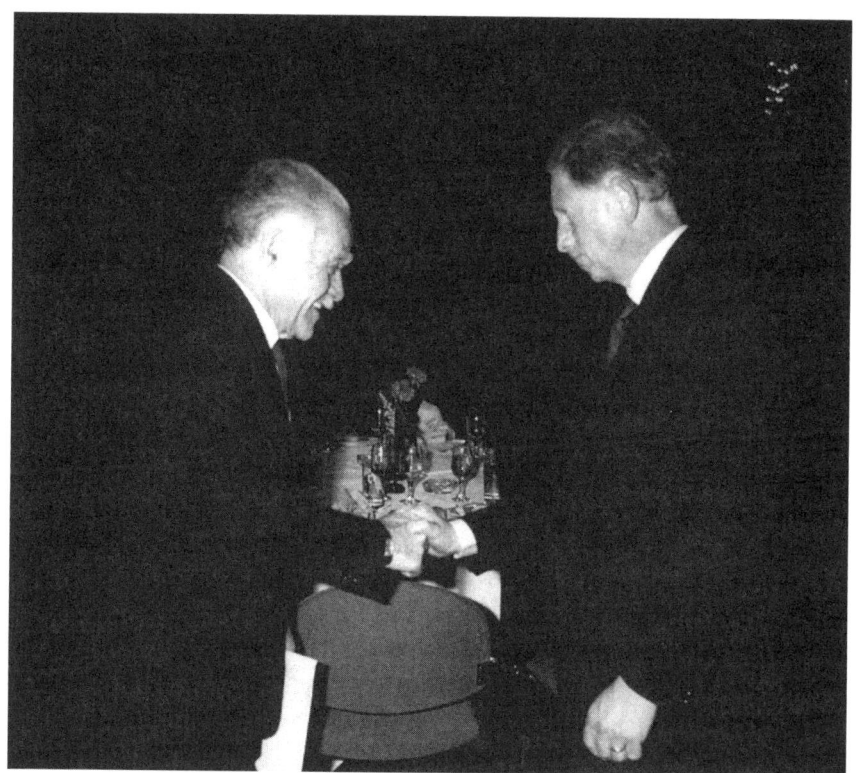

(above) With former Prime Minister of Israel, Yitzhak Shamir, at an Israeli state dinner in Jerusalem

(left) Personal birthday greeting from Chaim Herzog during his presidency of Israel, 1988

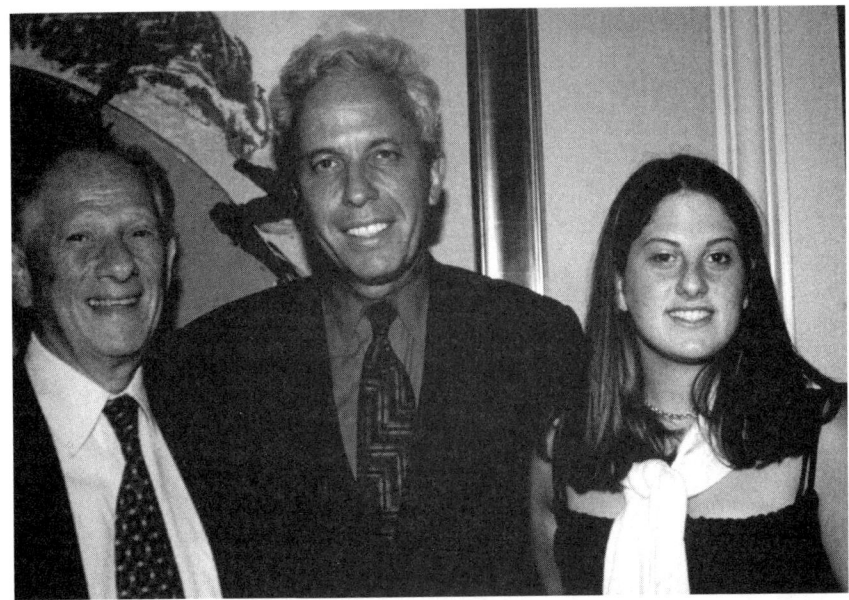

With New York City mayoral candidate Mark Green and my daughter Jessica at Denise Rich's apartment in Manhattan

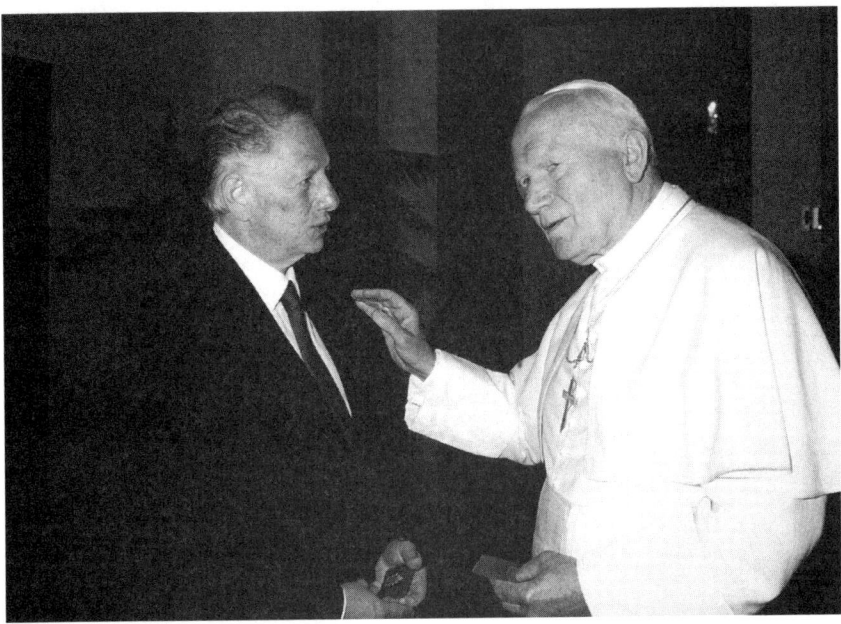

Photograph from my audience with Pope John Paul II at the Apostolic Palace, 1996

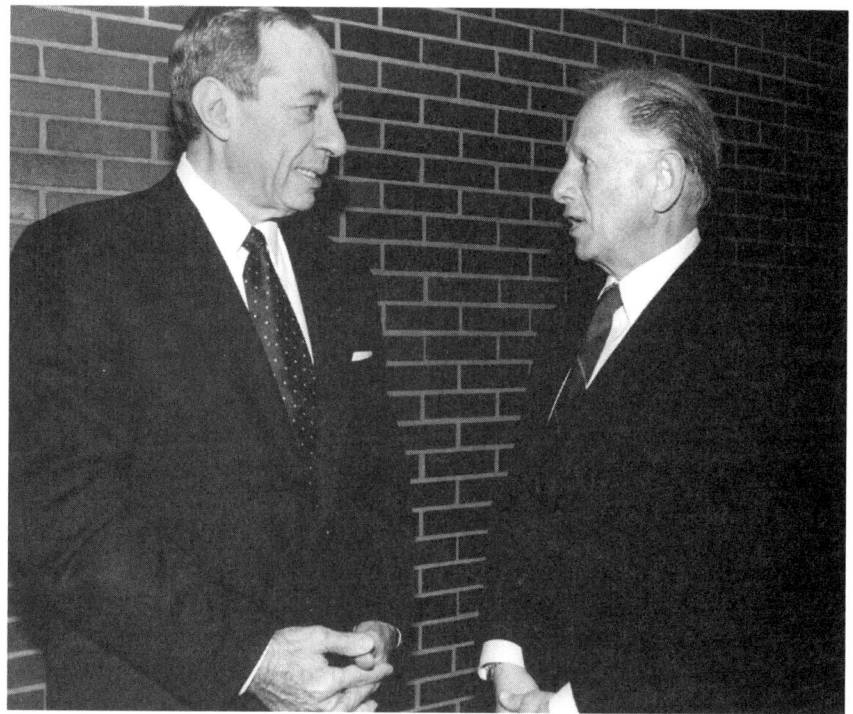

With former New York Governor Mario Cuomo at a Democratic fund raiser

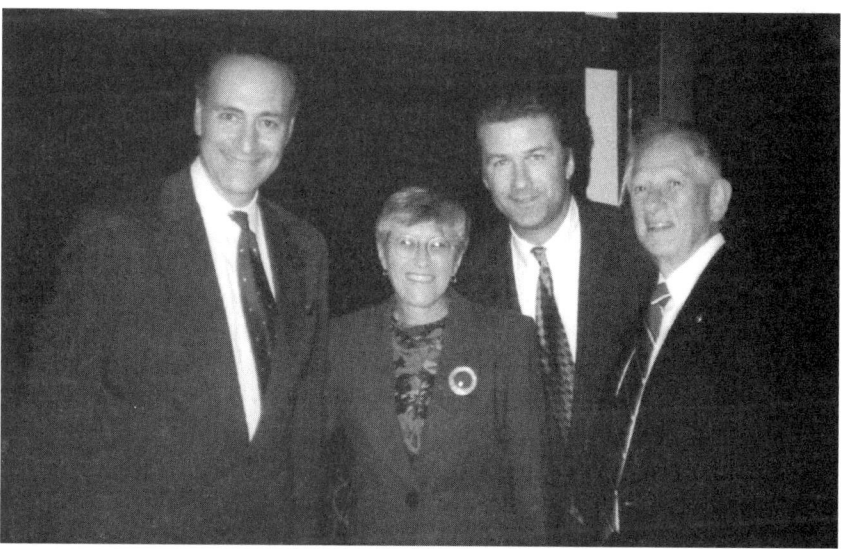

Left to right: Senator Chuck Schumer, Polly Rothman, Alec Baldwin and me at a private meeting for women's reproductive rights

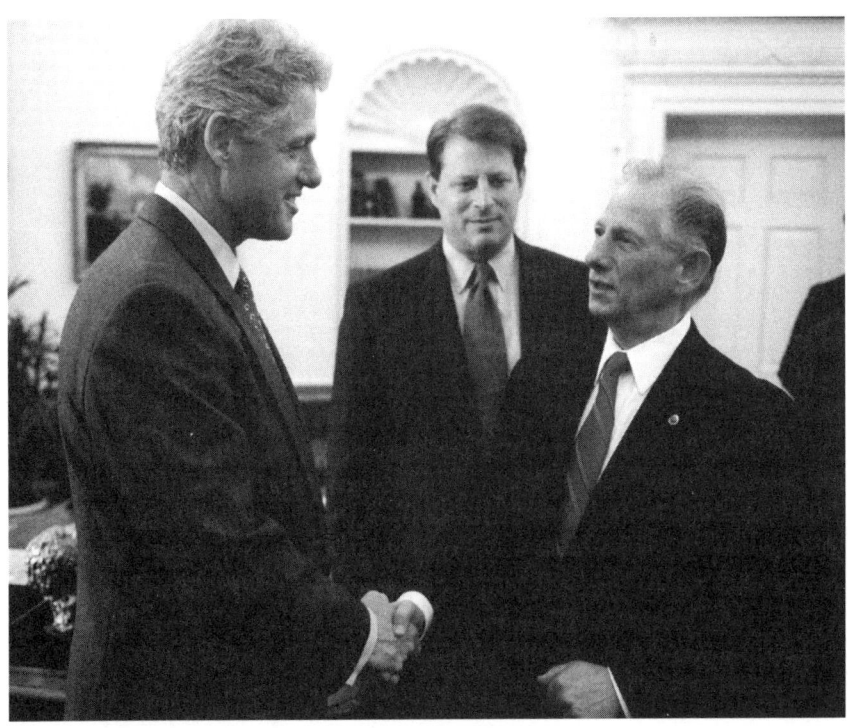

With President Clinton and Vice President Gore during my run for Congress in New York's 19th District in 1996

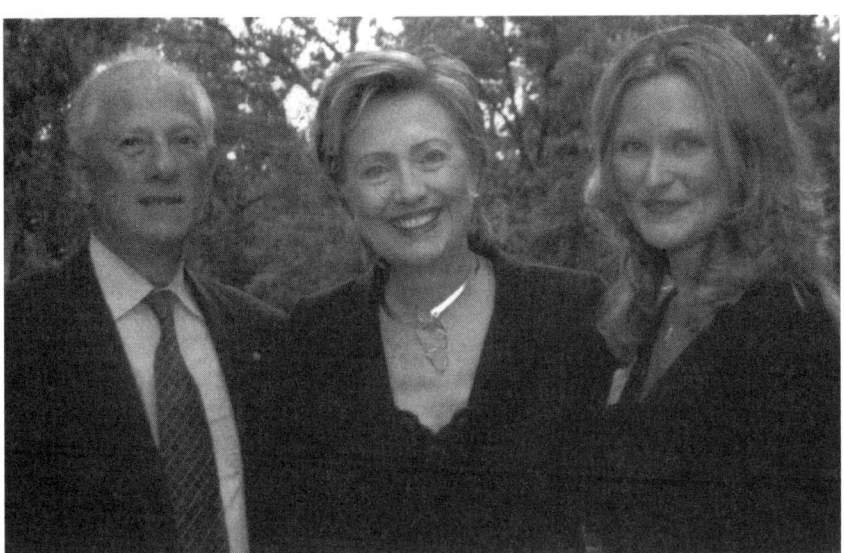

My wife Caryn and I pose with Hillary Clinton

ראש הממשלה
PRIME MINISTER

Jerusalem, September 21, 1992.
217-2

Dear Dr. Klein

Thank you for your very warm wishes of congratulation and words of support.

While there are many challenges ahead, I am optimistic that during this government's term in office significant progress will be made in the peace process and that the groundwork for a permanent settlement will be reached.

If my schedule permits, I look forward to meeting with you during your next visit to Israel.

With best regards,

Sincerely yours,

Y. Rabin
Yitzhak Rabin

Dr. Richard S. Klein, Chairman
State of Israel Bonds, Westchester, N. Y.
Yorktown Commons
1872 Commerce Street
Yorktown Heights, NY 10598

Letter from Prime Minister Yitzhak Rabin in recognition of my service during two Arab-Israeli wars, issued soon after he assumed office in 1992. Rabin was Head of General Staff of the Israeli Defense Forces when they reunified the city of Jerusalem in 1967.

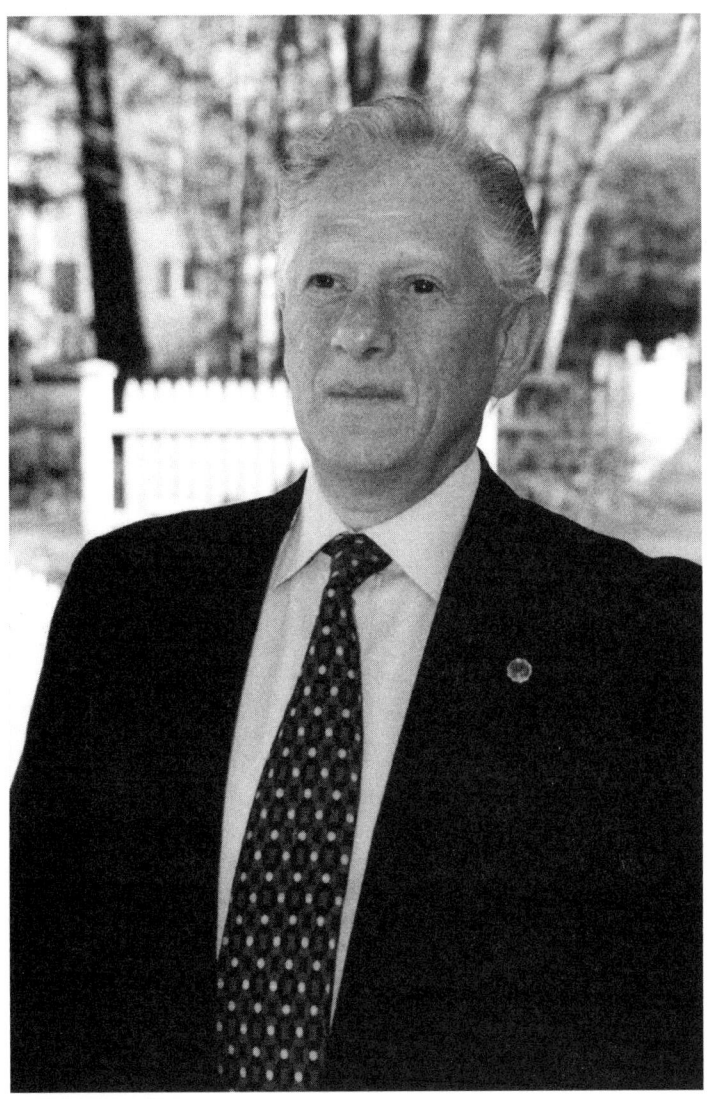

Publicity shot from my campaign for Congress

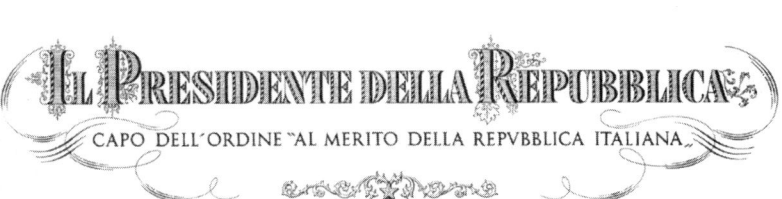

IL PRESIDENTE DELLA REPUBBLICA

CAPO DELL'ORDINE "AL MERITO DELLA REPUBBLICA ITALIANA"

In considerazione di particolari benemerenze;
Sentita la Giunta dell'Ordine al Merito della Repubblica Italiana
Sulla proposta del Presidente del Consiglio dei Ministri;
con Decreto in data Roma, 2 giugno 2001

HA CONFERITO

l'onorificenza di *Cavaliere*

al Dott. **Richard Klein**

con facoltà di fregiarsi delle insegne stabilite per tale classe.
Il Cancelliere dell'Ordine Al Merito della Repubblica Italiana è
incaricato dell'esecuzione del presente Decreto che sarà registrato alla Cancelleria
dell'Ordine medesimo.

FIRMATO *Ciampi*   CONTROFIRMATO *Amato*

Il Cancelliere dell'Ordine dichiara che in esecuzione delle Presidenziali
disposizioni

il Dott. Richard Klein

è stato iscritto nell'Elenco dei Cavalieri Est.   al N° 1680   Serie IV

IL CANCELLIERE DELL'ORDINE

IL DIRETTORE CAPO UFFICIO
DELLA CANCELLERIA

Certificate from the president of Italy conferring upon me the title of *Cavaliere,*
the highest level of knighthood open to a civilian who is not a citizen of Italy

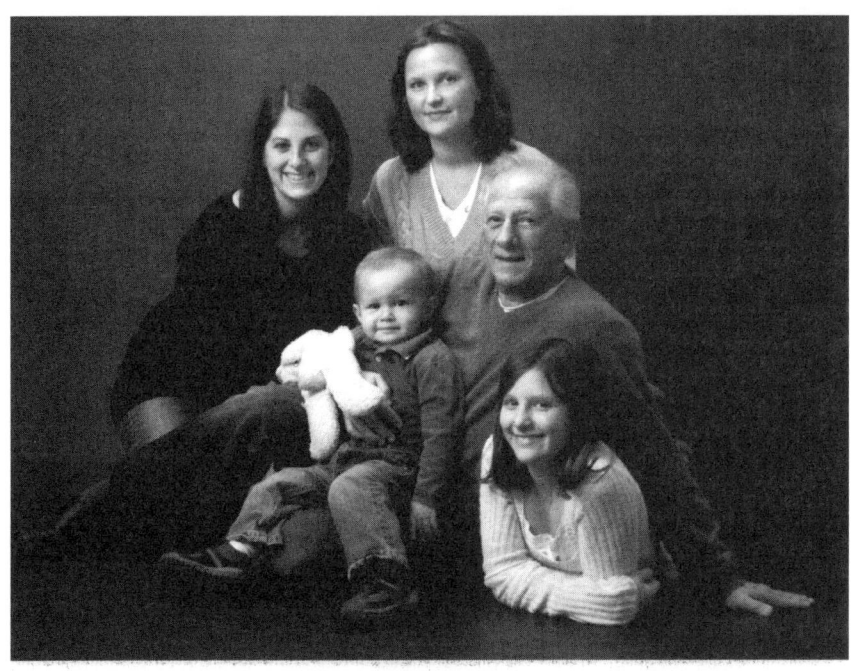

My family: daughter Jessica *(upper left)*, wife Caryn *(upper right)*, step daughter Arianna *(bottom right)* and my new son Matthew with "Mr. Puppie"

Traveling Through Life

In the introduction to this section, I used the device of comparing life to a journey—specifically, a train journey. Perhaps because the notion of a journey by train has a romantic element to it (think "Orient Express"). Perhaps because the idea of train travel calls to mind a simpler, "homier" time for some. Tangential to that, perhaps it is because I can still remember when long-distance journeys by train were quite common. And let me tell those of you who think that train travel could never measure up to the experience of flight that you simply do not understand what you are missing. True that a plane will always get you there faster, but a train journey is unparalleled in offering the traveler a chance to see parts of America, or any other country, that one would not normally get to see. It also gives a sense of progress as you take in the scenery and terrain through which you pass on the way to your destination.

Though I've already made this point in the introduction (which I have, in turn, referenced just one paragraph above), I'd like to further the analogy by transferring the focus from the mode of transport for our "journey" to the other "passengers" that are with us on the ride. During our journey through life, people get on and off our trains, and we can't always control when or where they get on or how long they will stay. Sometimes there are those that we don't want to get off: a lost love; a friend, relative, or even parent with whom we've had an irreparable break; perhaps someone whom life has simply taken from us way too soon. Sometimes, though, there are those we want to leave. Perhaps they've brought more baggage then the train can safely handle, causing it to slow down, drag, and occasionally even derail.

• • •

There are people that enter our lives who turn out to be bad influences. I don't mean in the sense of the brooding hoodlum mainstay of the after school special and countless *Bad News Bears* movies. What I do mean is the type of person who always seems to have a depressive effect on those around him (or her). Whether a result of their own insecurities, unresolved anger issues, a certain sense of self-loathing, or any other emotional or social shortcoming, these folks always seem to be able to spread their bad moods, personal discomfort and dissatisfactions to those closest to them. I have found that, when left to our own devices, we are all quite capable of making ourselves feel lonely, sad, and depressed, the entrée to poor mental and physical well-being. Willingly spending time with people who emotionally drag you down to their level of daily misery is not only unhealthy, it borders on crazy.

When he was in his nineties, Bob Hope used to say: "I only hang with "up" people. That's how I made it so far." For some reason, there was one day that his quote really drove things home to me. Obviously my profession had long ago taught me that life is precarious, that we can be hale and hearty one day and have disaster strike the next. But it was only then that it dawned on me just how many minute factors come to bear on the quality of life beyond basic physical health. With that mini revelation, it seemed foolish for me, or for anyone, not to take charge of as many of those extra factors as possible. As the old saying goes, life is not a dress rehearsal.

So when I closed in on age 60, I made a decision to reevaluate all of my personal relationships. I considered all the people with whom maintaining a relationship and sharing my life meant nothing more than a frustrating and one-sided struggle of ignored phone calls and invitations that were often deferred and never reciprocated. I made note of all those who were unshakeable in their belief that they knew everything about everything, and always felt compelled to make the breadth and depth of their "knowledge" a public matter, sure that any evidence contrary to their theories or positions was evidence of some sort of conspiracy of willful ignorance on the part of the world at large. I made a list in my head of my acquaintances that regularly dispensed unhappiness, tension, selfishness, or arguments into their interactions with me and with others. And I made it a point to cut them out of my life.

In the year before Arthur Ashe died of AIDS-related complications, Arthur's wife Jeanne made it a point to keep anyone who could have made Arthur sad or unhappy away from their home and out of their lives. I'm certain that, as few in number as his final days were, there were that many more of them thanks to her decision. Like Arthur

Ashe, we can't always foresee the mishaps and illnesses that may befall us or our loved ones. But we can take charge of our happiness in an effort to prevent "infection" from the bad vibes and negative attitudes of others.

• • •

So sometimes we lose fellow travelers from our "train" too soon, and other times we have to force people off. Either way, the train continues on from one station to the next, with or without our consent, chugging along at speeds that are just as out of our control as are its list of passengers. When we're younger, the drag of time seems interminably slow and we consume ourselves with anticipation for the day when we can put youth behind us and take our places in the adult world, where for some reason we think we'll never again have to listen to the dictates of another. Of course, once we reach that point many of us begin to reconsider. But by then we realize that the months and years seem to be whizzing by at an ever increasing pace, that there may be more of the journey behind us than ahead.

It helps to have a plan, a "map," if you will, to aid us as we navigate through this voyage. If we are going to enjoy the journey, we can and should have some say as to which route our train is going to take. Not a rigid travel plan that depends on maintaining a rigid schedule at all costs, just an aid that reminds us to look for certain signposts as we make our trip through life as best we can. And we need to be prepared to overcome hazards along the way and understand that, if lucky, we're in this for "the long haul." And like any long haul, we don't sprint but pace ourselves, neither too fast nor too slow, sure of breath and with steady stride. For we need to keep in mind that the very point of this trip is not necessarily the destination, but enjoying the voyage on the way. Or as Willa Cather put it in *O Pioneers!* nearly a century ago, "The road is all …"

The most common of these "maps" for most of us are our dreams and ambitions. Whether harbored since youth or stumbled upon at some random point in life, it is these ideals and goals that give the voyage of our lives shape and meaning. As we strive to achieve them, both our actions toward our dreams and the dreams themselves take on added and deeper meanings and end up enriching our lives by the lessons they teach us, both in victory and in failure. Is the attainment of our ultimate goal a worthy end in itself if it requires the sacrifice of something held dear? Or the forsaking of opportunities that may lead us down divergent and unforeseen, but perhaps equally enriching, paths? Conversely, is failure (except perhaps in the most extreme and vital of circumstances) a reason to give up on hopes and dreams in general, or even on life itself? Personal experience has taught me that the answer to each question is "no." But each one of you will have to answer those questions for yourselves, and perhaps you will arrive at answers that are different from mine. But that's the beauty of it.

Unfortunately, many people try to take short cuts instead of fulfilling life's ambitions, settling for what can be easily achieved or acquired rather than what they really desire. By doing so, I feel we help derail our very own train. Some of the starkest examples of this that I have personally witnessed involved co-workers in the medical profession. I have encountered more than one person, male and female, who set their sights on becoming a doctor or registered nurse (RN), only to stop at the level of practical nurse (more formally, "licensed practical nurse," or LPN) simply because it offered the path of least resistance, one to two years, as opposed to a minimum of two years to become an RN, and more to become an MD. Though there is often a sense of benign rivalry between doctors and nurses, it was usually these few LPNs that seemed to harbor a tangible sense of resentment against doctors and RNs alike. It was as if they had convinced themselves that doctors and RNs radiated smug superiority by dint of having gone to school for a few more years, and had decided to lord it over them specifically. That they were at times unpleasant work partners goes without saying, but I can't help but wonder where all that anger and frustration goes when the work day ends.

Let me make clear that there is much pride and glory in being a practical nurse, and there are many reasons why people aspire to that level as an end in itself. In America's universally overworked, generally understaffed, and frequently underappreciated hospitals and clinics, they are vital links in the chain that keeps things functioning. The example was specific to certain individuals, and the point is that one can go the distance if one really wants to, and might end up miserable if too afraid or lazy to follow through. If you do find yourself in such a situation, it is never, ever too late to take charge and take the plunge. Desire, belief in yourself, and a healthy amount of effort can take you as far as your dreams will allow.

Remember, if you don't take control of your own train, you're just going along for the ride. And though it may not be convenient or cheap or easy to do, most things of real value never are.

PART 3
THINGS

Introduction

FOREIGN CULTURES, THE INTRICACIES OF FAITH, the depth and breadth of the human mind—as inscrutable as any or all of these may be for some, the world of medicine can seem just as byzantine and impenetrable to the uninitiated. Maybe that's why television shows like *Quincy, ER, CSI,* and the like are so popular and so long-lived. The everyday world of medicine generates more than enough fodder for both screen writers and mystery buffs with its seemingly endless false leads, hidden clues, and complex yet often invisible network of relationships, causes, and effects, each leading down a series of potential blind alleys.

As an example, I'm put in mind of a building from my *alma mater,* the University of Rome. Near the ancient campus compound, there is a large and impressive building to the immediate right. It bears the name "The Institute for Syphilis and Dermatology."

Interesting combination, no? What could the link possibly be between dermatology and history's most famous venereal disease? The pairing cracks open the door to any number of jokes, but the fact that it is carved above the entrance to a departmental building at one of the oldest institutions of higher learning in the Western world leaves many scratching their heads.

Before the antibiotic era, when syphilis was rampant, the rashes caused by this disease were plentiful and diverse beyond the initial skin ulcerations in the genital area. Therefore the presentation of any rash or skin lesion always contained syphilis as part of the differential diagnosis; it was so prevalent that it deserved equal billing with dermatology. Even during my training in the early 1960s, we still saw the many different varieties of skin rashes that were the results of syphilis, as well as malformations in babies born to sufferers, and even elderly people with telltale signs of prior disease. I once examined, as part of a supervised group of medical students, an elderly grandmother suffering from bronchitis when the professor pointed out very quietly that one pupil was pin-point while the other was dilated, a sign of late-stage neurological syphilis. There was something in her past that certainly no one would want to talk about to her grandchildren.

Syphilis in its tertiary stage also causes changes in personality and dementia. It has long been rumored that Idi Amin, the ruthless former dictator of Uganda, was treated for neurological syphilis in Israel while there for a military training course, long before the fateful raid on Entebbe. Though never proven, he was known to have a taste for brothels and was treated for "social diseases" several times as a young man in the British Colonial Army. Perhaps tertiary syphilis was the reason he was so crazy.

I have taken this detour through the wonderful world of syphilis to illustrate the number of hidden rooms and secret passages in the great labyrinth of medicine, and how so many seemingly unrelated things are somehow connected. Since I've already introduced you to some of the "People" with whom I've crossed paths, and taken you to some of the more interesting "Places" I've been (and shared the lessons I've learned from all of them along the way), I'd like to teach you all a few "Things" about practical medicine and health maintenance, some more straight-ahead scientific, some philosophical, some coldly practical, but all guaranteed to maintain your interest. I really do feel, as I said in the first section, that the modern doctor-patient relationship should be more of a partnership and less of a dictatorship. To that end, I am quite glad to see my patients becoming more informed about certain things, thanks to the Internet and sites such as WebMD.

But there's a lot more out there than what can be found on WebMD, and some things will be worth finding while others should be ignored or taken with the proper number of salt grains. Almost every day the news blares mixed messages from some new medical report or another, resulting in a huge spate of patient visits just so they can come to me and complain, "I thought dairy was good, now the surgeon general tells me it's bad. Which is it, doc?"

This is where knowledge of some medical basics as well as of yourself can help you. When consulting medical journals or popular websites, it is important to assess the information in the proper context and work out a solution that feels right for you. In a way, it's a review and reinforcement of what I said before: our body can usually tell us when something is wrong. I'd like to hope that this third section will help us listen to our bodies as closely as we do (or should) our doctors. Think of it as a limited crash course of study through medical school.

Now, class, turn the page and we'll begin ...

You Can Be Whatever You Want, Just Will It and Do It with a Smile

So just how shocked are you at the way this man of science has introduced so many patently unscientific elements to this collection of anecdotes about medicine? Luck, chance, faith, I believe that all of these have played some part, sometimes small, sometimes not, in all of our lives and careers. And though I believe in the power and validity of all of these things (to an extent), I will admit the fact that they contain more than a bit of the indefinable and mysterious is offputting for some people. And I can easily understand that. But there is a tangent to all of these, perhaps a corollary or a common foundation, that is the pared-down essence of all the factors I have mentioned: the ability to maintain a positive outlook.

Sometimes this most simple of things can seem like the most herculean task when things seem the darkest. When health problems or other challenges touch your life, it's easy to go numb, to become disconnected, to just feel like giving up. You feel as if you have just experienced some sort of grand existential betrayal, and the immediate impulse is to lay blame, to judge yourself or those closest to you (often quite harshly), and become angry and resentful. Sometimes I second-guess my personal feelings about things like faith and luck in reference to this issue. If we are taught and/or fervently believe that some outside power or entity has a say over or potential effect upon our futures and happiness, how can we keep a positive, healthy attitude in the face of God or the Fates or what have you obviously demonstrating to us that we have somehow fallen out of favor and will pay a dear price for having done so?

This is a fundamentally flawed but widely accepted view of life. Though I still believe in the positive power of both faith and luck, neither, in my mind, is an absolute. Both have great power for good, I do not consider them be-alls and end-alls. There is an old Hassidic parable that says "The Holy One, blessed be He, is our shield and our salvation, our protector and provider, and He is with us in all places and at all times. But only a fool willingly bares his neck for the sword while simply reasoning that the Name (of God) will protect him." Put another, more succinct way, God helps those who help themselves; and feel free to substitute "fortune favors the bold" for the previous, if you are so inclined.

• • •

One evening in the summer before I entered medical school, when I was working as an emergency ambulance attendant for Long Island Jewish Hospital, my response team was called to a house where a young girl had attempted suicide by overdosing with pills. We did our best to stabilize her condition and put her into the ambulance to get her to the emergency room.

While in transit, she told me about the problems that had driven her to attempt suicide. She told me she was having difficulty finding friends, getting a job, making any progress in her life. On top of which, she was extremely insecure about her weight. She was actually quite obese, a situation made even more pointed by the fact that she lived with her very attractive sister. I almost felt guilty then. My dreams were coming together at that time in my life, and here I was confronted with someone at the other polar extreme of life. In an effort to reach out to her, I told her my motto: believe and you can achieve.

We got her to the hospital in plenty of time. She was admitted, treated, and that was the last I heard of her ... until one year later. I was working the summer after my first year of medical school in Rome, again at Long Island Jewish, when a young, pretty, shapely woman came into the emergency room and sought me out. I had no idea who she was until she reminded me of that night the previous year. She was the obese girl who had attempted suicide on my watch. She said her life turned around because of that night and what I had said.

The truth is you are the one with the most power over your life. This doesn't mean you can control every external circumstance or illness that befalls you, but it does mean that you can determine your response to and attitudes about them. And this ultimately determines your mental and emotional state, which informs your actions and decisions and, finally, transforms your condition. It's natural to feel sad, even some self-pity, when things aren't going your way; it is even more understandable when you suffer a serious illness or personal setback. And it's okay to allow this emptiness, this "dark night of the soul" to occur, because these feelings are a natural part of the coping process.

But just because it's natural doesn't mean it's constructive. A tornado is "natural," but you wouldn't want to live inside one. Similarly, though whatever negativity you feel may be eminently understandable, it will quickly end up working against you. Whatever we focus on tends to expand to fill all the available space in our lives. If, while suffering from an illness, you focus only on your condition and discomfort and a sense of hopelessness and victimhood, it is the illness that ends up mastering you while dashing whatever hopes you may have for recovery. If you face a life obstacle or setback and focus upon it to the detriment of all else, it becomes an anchor around your neck. The condition from which you suffer, in a sense, becomes who you are, steals your identity, and may end up getting the final victory by defining your image for others after the battle is over, whether it ends up being won or lost. If you give more attention to whatever *is* working beyond the immediate situation, things have a chance of reaching a better conclusion because, on one small level, you've already achieved a sort of victory by not letting your situation define you. Put another way, what you appreciate tends to appreciate.

Many, many years ago, before I even applied to medical school, I was seriously dating a girl named Joan from northern Queens. We were very much in love, and I looked forward to her being around in my life in that amorphous way that young people of that age have when they are engaged in affairs of the heart. So imagine how I felt when Joan told me she was breaking up with me. She had to, she said, because her mom was forcing her hand. It seems that Joan's mother didn't think I would ever amount to anything, and she insisted that her daughter stop wasting her time.

About two years after that, the same year, as a matter of fact, that the young woman who had attempted suicide sought me out after her transformation., I was working my ambulance attendant job at Long Island Jewish Hospital after my first year of medical school when we got another attempted suicide call. But this time the address of the call rang a bell and got my heart racing with terrible anxiety. It was Joan's house.

It turned out that it was not Joan, but her mother who had attempted suicide by ingesting a large amount of disinfectant. We arrived to find her doubled over in agony, her mouth and face stained a deep purple by the solution she had consumed. As we labored to save her life (which we did, by the way), I could not help but be stricken by the irony of the fact that I was not only on my way to becoming a doctor and realizing my dreams, but was even now working to save the life of a woman who didn't think I would ever "amount to anything."

• • •

At some point, regardless of how bad the situation may be, you must find something to be grateful for. Not just outside of your crisis but right smack in the middle of it. That darkness you are experiencing is the light in potential just as the dark, rich soil is new life in potential. Ask yourself, "What benefits am I (or my family) getting from this problem? How will I be better, stronger, or wiser because of it?" The answers may not come easily, but eventually you'll begin to see that silver lining. And as you become grateful for it, your "curse" will yield its blessings.

I'm sure that many of those reading these words will respond to my above prescription for a positive attitude with something along the lines of "easier said than done, doc." Fair enough, and quite so. For many of us, such a reaction is neither first nor second nor third nature. Indeed, the very idea of such a show of courage or defiance in the face of potentially crushing adversity is practically inconceivable for most of us. This ability is what causes people to make divisions among themselves according to certain character traits that end up stamping some with the label of "hero." But history has shown us that anyone has the potential for heroism. From Joan of Arc to Elie Weisel to Ryan White—the young boy who became a symbol of the deadly reach of AIDS in that disease's early days, and ended up becoming a living synonym for dignity and courage in the face of fear, misunderstanding, and ignorance—all of these people, and many who fell in between, were simple people forced into extraordinary and complex circumstances, and who rose above these circumstances by remaining simple, honest, and true to themselves. I cannot speak to the innate abilities of strangers, but I would like each and every one of you to file that little bit of information away if the day ever comes when you are put to the test.

And though the above is more than a little gloomy, this is probably the most advantageous time to remind all of you that one of the most effective tools in this morbid battle is humor. (And just in time, too. I can imagine readers everywhere throwing down this book in depression, frustration, and fear after the last few pages to seek solace in the bottle of their choice.)

Though I briefly addressed this topic earlier in my discussion of my patient Benny, I understand that this is counterintuitive for some, especially when things look their worst. "How can you make jokes at a time like this?" is a common phrase in such situations; but it's not about jokes, per se, or what we think of as jokes. Too many people, when faced with such a situation or even when just contemplating one, immediately think of the small-minded, mean-spirited type of jokes, as if it were appropriate to give a grievously ill person a "hot foot" or make them the butt of some sort of practical joke. Instead, it's all about sharing emotion to relieve a greater emotional burden. We can sympathize with a patient, sometimes we can even empathize, but no one can ever fully understand another individual's uniquely personal experience. Humor is a way to bridge a divide, to reach out and connect with someone when they may need it the most. Rather than demean the seriousness of life, in these situations humor makes life more palatable.

When I was a young student still in Infectious Disease training, my mentor was a brilliant physician whose clinical and diagnostic skills were practically awe-inspiring. In nearly every way imaginable, he was an ideal medical role model. But he utterly lacked the ability to share or understand a patient's emotion. He thought my joking with seriously ill patients was a waste of time at best, and perhaps even cruel. Not only was it unfathomable for him that a terminally ill patient would have the time or desire for some light-hearted humor, it was as if my attempt at distraction for these poor people was beyond my mission as a doctor. Despite his academic and scientific brilliance, he simply could not grasp how humor offered a release of unfocused anxieties and tension, bringing both the patient and the physician closer and helping to divert the doom and gloom of the sickroom. While it may not have the curative powers of chemotherapy or the duration of a time-release pill, humor can lighten a mood, dull the pain, or brighten a face quicker than any other medicine known to man.

Besides being a salve in desperate times, humor can also be a tonic that corrects a situation before it becomes too dire. Such was the case for "Rosa,"[8] a sensitive young woman with a strict, old-world immigrant father and a long history of depression. By the time she was in her early twenties she had two serious suicide attempts under her belt. The last attempt left her hospitalized for three weeks.

As it happened, Rosa was in the pre-med program at her college and had been accepted to the very same medical school I had attended at the University of Rome. She was excited by the opportunity to pursue her dream in the old country of her parents' stories, as well as the chance to get out from under the watchful eye of her father, who was himself quite proud that his little girl would be studying medicine at *La Sapienza* ("Wisdom," the familiar nickname of the school in Italian). One day she came in crying, telling me that she was going to kill herself because she failed an extradisciplinary senior class in college, which meant that she wouldn't graduate and therefore would not be able to go to medical school. I called her college president, then her dean, and ultimately her course instructor. I explained that I was her family physician and that, given her history, she would definitely attempt to kill herself, and asked if there was some way out of the situation that was acceptable to all the parties involved. They all met and subsequently changed her grade from "F" to "D". Rosa thus graduated.

One year later, she called me from Rome. This didn't necessarily surprise me, as I tend to forge personal relationships with many of my patients (as you would know if you'd been paying attention from the first section), but it soon became evident that all was not well for Rosa. I am a bit hazy on the details now, but it seems that she was having another bout of severe depression. Perhaps her newfound independence or her unfamiliar surroundings were overwhelming for her, perhaps the program at the university was more of a challenge than she had bargained for. Whatever the trigger for her depressive episode, it was obviously full upon her and she was again contemplating suicide. But this time my opportunities to help were limited. Not only was I unable to gauge the cause of her depression, but we were separated by an ocean and the better part of a continent.

---

8 Not her real name.

I was worried because I knew what Rosa was capable of when it came to doing herself real, immediate harm. Realizing that I had few options available, I did what came naturally and tried to diffuse the situation with a little light-hearted but well placed absurdity. "Rosa," I said, "after all I went through for you to get you out of Westchester and into the university, if you commit suicide I'm going to go over there and kill you myself!" We both paused then; for a brief, horrifying moment, I wasn't sure if she understood what I was doing. It was one of those instances when a moment seems to drag on into eternity, but it couldn't have been more than one or two seconds at the most before she started laughing hysterically. With that, her mood seemed to lift enough for her pull out of her depressive tailspin and concentrate on living her life rather than wanting to end it. It has been some time since she and I last spoke, but I know through common friends and acquaintances that she has managed to do very well for herself in the intervening years. And all because of my sparkling wit.

O.K., not really. But I'd like to think I've made my point. If you are willing to inject a little humor, lightheartedness, and loving fun into the lives of those who are sick or dying or simply need it, you may not help heal their physical problem but you'll almost always uplift their heavy heart and weary spirit.

That Mind Game Can Get in the Way

I**N THE FIRST SECTION OF THIS BOOK**, I discussed how people will accept nearly any physical diagnosis at face value but tend to balk when told their problems may be psychological in nature. It's practically a truism: folks will go running to a heart surgeon ready to undergo a transplant that very day if they even get the impression that this is what their physician is telling them to do. But tell them they may have a serious psychological problem and the hemming and hawing begins, because there couldn't *possibly* be anything wrong with them. After all, that would mean they're crazy, and they're certainly not crazy.

But sometimes our psyche gets the last laugh. Or at least gets a chance to use the body to let off a little steam of its own.

Barbara was a 25-year-old nurse who usually came in for a physical once a year. One day she came in very agitated, complaining about having shortness of breath. I quickly noticed her self-diagnosis was at odds with her physical appearance: she wasn't panting or in any major distress and she didn't seem uncomfortable or unduly anxious. When asked to describe the sensation, she said she felt as if she didn't take in enough air when she took a deep breath, and had to take another and another. Her lungs didn't feel as if they were filling up enough. After a thorough examination I could find nothing wrong, and told her so. She was reassured and off she went.

The next week Barbara showed up again, this time complaining of heart palpitations. Her heart felt as if it were skipping beats, she explained, most often while she was watching TV or reading a book or relaxing, but never while she was exerting herself or exercising. Again, a thorough evaluation turned up everything as normal and she was once again reassured and sent home. Barbara returned for a third time the following week. This time she said she felt as if there was an obstruction or tightening of her throat, almost as if something was stuck behind her Adam's apple, choking her (and, yes, women do have Adam's apples).

At this point, I changed my approach from the clinical to the personal. There is a fairly common anxiety-provoked syndrome called *globus hystericus* which is defined as a sensation of a lump in the throat experienced during "hysteria," which itself is defined as "a psychoneurosis marked by emotional excitability and disturbances of the psychic, sensory, ... and visceral functions without an organic basis." The tightening of the throat, the heart palpitations, the feeling of not taking in enough air with each breath, all of these complaints combined with the utter lack of any real physical symptoms told me more was going on here than met the eye.

I asked her what was going on in her life. There had to be a reason that a patient I was used to seeing once a year for a routine check-up had now come in three times in as many weeks with detailed complaints but with no signs of anything wrong. She looked puzzled at my question and said, rather noncommittally, "Nothing ... really." Knowing better, I waited a beat before she finally admitted, as if it was a mere afterthought, "Oh, I am getting married next month. I've been busy making arrangements." Somehow, this trained medical professional couldn't see the connection between a very stressful time and a sudden increase in classic stress-related complaints.

Sadly, this is more common than you might think. It's very common for patients to have these multiple psychosomatic episodes prior to a significant life event. When I was studying for an exam to help me transfer from medical school in Italy to one in New York, I wound up in the local emergency room one evening with palpitations. I thought I was having a heart attack at the age of twenty four. The E.R. physician asked if anything was happening in my life that would be causing anxiety and I sincerely answered no. Though a medical student, even I couldn't catch the connection. Sometimes it happens during a divorce, or a parent or child's major illness, or it can occur three or four months after a catastrophe, like some kind of mental or physical "delayed reaction." The body usually coasts along during the emergencies; responding as it should, but it is during the cooling-off period, usually three months later, when things begin to finally break down.

A patient named Mary came in with a complaint of her hair falling out. Unfortunate for anyone, but more so for a woman, and especially for her; Mary was a very attractive woman for whom hair was an important part of her beauty and allure. She was quite unnerved dur-

ing the examination, and asked and opined about the possible causes of her condition. Perhaps it was a glandular or hormonal problem?
No, because any glandular or hormonal problem would present with
other symptoms besides hair loss, and she showed none of them.
Maybe she was experiencing an early and extreme menopause?
Unlikely, because menopause, at early or regular onset, also presents
with a host of symptoms, and though many women experience some
hair loss as they get older, it is almost always gradual and rarely
immediately related to the natural process of menopause. There was,
however, a condition called stress alopecia that was characterized by
massive hair loss due to some sort of physical or emotional shock.
Had she, I asked, suffered a severe physical or emotional trauma
recently? She hadn't been in any sort of car wreck or suffered any
physical injury, she hadn't suddenly discontinued taking birth control pills (the sudden change in hormone levels that results can often
cause some short-term hair loss) ... no, she couldn't think of any
stressor that would cause her hair to fall out. She said that she had
been tending to her father for the better part of the past year as he
battled cancer, a battle he had sadly lost just a few months earlier, but
it couldn't have possibly had anything to do with that.

Or could it?

She then told me what the last year had been like for her. Her
father's diagnosis was a complete shock, and the cancer had him in
and out of hospitals for months. Through it all, she had behaved like
a trooper, visiting him daily at this or that hospital and taking him
for his weekly chemotherapy treatments when he was discharged. But
she didn't have any signs of anxiety during all that time. I explained
to her that it's common for people to "break down" after the pro-
tracted illness, when the stressor has been eliminated and their body
or mind no longer has to focus on the crisis and finally has time to
return its concentration back to them. It was not unlike Barbara's
heart palpitations, which were reactions to anxiety but which only
bothered her when her body or mind were trying to rest. When physically active or consciously tackling a challenge, the mind is focused
on mastering the task at hand. When we are at rest, the mind has a
chance to stand back and consider all the problems we have been facing. The problems cause us undue anxiety, which causes release of
adrenaline, causing our hearts to react with either a quickened pulse
or skipped beats.

Fortunately, neither Barbara's nor Mary's problems were harmful or permanent. Once her body and mind had a chance to process the shock of her father's ordeal and unfortunate death, Mary's hair loss ceased and the hair eventually began to grow back. As for Barbara, she is now happily married and she and her husband are in the process of building their first home.

Be alert to, but not paranoid of, the body's subtle messages that the mind may be in a period of transition or flux, and take them for what they are: messages that your body and mind are trying to work something out in tandem. There are even simple remedies for some of these anxiety-related symptoms that are effective and drug-free. My friend Basil, one of the happiest, most upbeat people I have ever met, occasionally suffers from something known as P.A.T. (paroxysmal atrial tachycardia) during periods of stress and anxiety. In healthy people, this is a harmless racing of the heart that causes no real problems. It wasn't serious or frequent enough in Basil's case to require preventative medications, but it was still something that bothered and frightened him. So I taught him how to return his heart to a normal rhythm through stimulating his sympathetic nervous system by rubbing the tops of the eyeballs, specifically the tiny notch in the upper orbital bone. I also introduced him to the magic of Valsalvering (the act of performing the Valsalva maneuver), which involves taking a deep breath and then trying to blow your nose but preventing air from coming out of the nostrils (the same action people take to adjust the pressure in their inner ears when flying or taking a train through a tunnel).

There are other common symptoms of anxiety that at first appear to be signs of serious trouble. More often than not though, the true source is mental rather than physical; and if your imagination has you dead on arrival at the doctor's office you're less likely to make that appointment in the first place. Take the time to rationally discuss these symptoms with your physician, and don't be afraid or ashamed to see a mental health professional if the situation seems to call for you to do so. Anxiety about the unknown is a normal mental reaction and occurs in all of us. If you remember that outside influences on your mental state can cause physical reactions and abnormal psychological responses, and you do an honest self-inquiry into the cause of your symptoms, you'll not only avoid unnecessary doctor visits, you'll also alleviate some of your anxiety-related symptoms.

Anxiety and Coping Mechanisms

Anxiety and fear are part of our lives. Feeling anxious is normal before some experiences, like walking down a dark street or before taking an exam, but this is actually good because it makes us more alert or careful. The problem arises when feelings of stress and anxiety persist. Symptoms of chronic, ongoing anxiety include: feeling restless, edgy, and keyed up, having trouble controlling these feelings, tiring easily, having trouble concentrating, irritability, increased muscle tension, sleeplessness, a feeling of butterflies in ones stomach, and a seeming pounding of the heart.

THE GENERALIZED ANXIETY DISORDER SELF-TEST

PART I—Yes or No:
- You experience feelings of excessive worry at least 50% of the time.
- You have difficulty controlling your worrying.
- You worry persistently for six months or more.

(One or more "yes" answers indicate unhealthy levels of anxiety.)

PART II—Yes or No:
- You often feel restless, keyed-up, or on edge.
- You tire quickly.
- You have problems concentrating.
- You are highly irritable.
- In addition to these feelings, you experience frequent muscle tension.
- You have trouble falling asleep or staying asleep, or restless and unsatisfying sleep.
- Your "normal" anxiety interferes with your daily life.

(Answering "yes" to three or more of these questions indicates anxiety.)

GENERAL TREATMENT AND COPING MECHANISMS

- Avoid alcohol, which can hide your symptoms and precipitate symptoms of depression.
- Reduce caffeine intake. Caffeine can make people jittery and anxious, and can inhibit a good night's sleep.
- Try to exercise. Even mild exercise, such as walking thirty minutes daily, may have a positive effect on anxiety by producing apomorphines.

- Practice breathing or relaxation techniques. Breathing properly can reduce heart rates, lower blood pressure, and diminish muscle aches and pains. Proper breathing also increases one's blood circulation. Check out yoga, meditation classes, martial arts classes, or get yourself a personal trainer.
- Set limits and learn to say "no." Trying to cram too much into one's day can sap your energy. Set priorities and do not over extend your list of daily activities.

When all else fails, please contact your health care specialist.

Following are some web sites with extremely helpful information. They provide access to articles, brochures and helpful activities.

American Psychiatric Association (APA)

www.healthyminds.org

Anxiety Disorders Association of America (ADAA)

www.adaa.org

Mental Health America

www.mentalhealthamerican.net

National Alliance on Mental Illness (NAMI)

www.nami.org

You Are What You Eat, So Watch What You Consume

AH, WHAT A MAGNIFICENT MACHINE IS THE HUMAN BODY. Every minute of every day it is sending us messages, some of which we hear and some of which we don't. Some of them we may not understand, but some are absolutely unmistakable.

Food poisoning is a pretty common occurrence and rarely life threatening. Depending on the type of food poisoning, symptoms can begin anywhere from a few hours to several days after eating contaminated food. The typical symptoms include abdominal pain, diarrhea, vomiting, and fever, though some forms of food poisoning will have vomiting without fever. And one of the most dangerous types, botulism, attacks the nervous system and leads to respiratory and musculoskeletal paralysis. Treatment of food poisoning, except botulism, deals mainly with preventing dehydration by putting back the fluids and electrolytes lost through vomiting and diarrhea, so a common remedy involves drinking plenty of Gatorade. In severe cases, though, a doctor may need to prescribe fluids intravenously.

We often think our homes are the last places that could possibly make us sick, but just as often our kitchens are the leading culprits. We often have our mothers or grandmothers or great-grandmothers whispering in our ears, literally or figuratively, as we make a favorite family dish that has been passed on from generation to generation. By all means, follow the recipe as diligently as possible. But hear your doctor whispering in your ear instead of grandma, and you'll spend more time in the kitchen and less in his office.

• • •

I have already established in other parts of this book how important certain rituals, beliefs, or traditions are to our sense of continuity, of belonging to a family or culture. This importance applies to rituals of the kitchen as much as those of worship or beliefs about health.

Because of this, changing them is often unthinkable, regardless of what common sense may say to the contrary.

For example, mushroom hunting was once a favorite pastime for people all across Europe. Even today people across the continent, from England to Italy to Russia, regularly go foraging in woods and fields as family groups, hunting parties, and young people on dates, hoping to find the wild, edible mushrooms that so many cultures consider a delicacy. Immigrants brought a love for this avocation to the new world, but the skills necessary to distinguish between a delicious oyster mushroom and a deadly panther cap toadstool went into serious decline with the rise in per capital personal income and the simultaneous advent of markets offering packaged foods, two factors that eliminated the need to go poking around the forest floor for sustenance. But the recent trend over the last few decades toward rediscovery of old ethnic traditions has led some to do as their great-grandparents did over a century ago and resume the hunt for the elusive wild mushroom. Unfortunately, while knowledge of the ritual may have survived, proper knowledge of the quarry has not always been passed town in tandem.

Case in point: I once got a phone call about an entire family that was terribly ill. I made a house call and found the mother, father, and four-teen-year-old son fighting each other to use the bathroom, each suffering from diarrhea, vomiting, or both. Meanwhile, in one corner sat their sixteen-year-old daughter, quiet, aloof, and obviously quite healthy.

I soon was able to glean the full story: the father had decided to make a batch of spaghetti sauce from scratch, and opted to make it truly authentic by picking mushrooms for the sauce from a nearby stand of woods. The evening it was to be served, the older daughter had disobeyed her parents by coming home late from school without calling first. Because of this transgression, she was punished with being forbidden to have dinner.

I had to admit the other three to the hospital for severe dehydration. She got to stay home alone and healthy. And with an empty house, I'm sure that she ate to her heart's content.

• • •

Toadstools are not ever meant to be eaten. But sometimes—quite often, really—food poisoning is the result of a safe, common, everyday food that has been improperly handled or prepared. One of the most common culprits is undercooked or uncooked animal protein. Rocky Balboa may have impressed a generation of young fitness buffs and bodybuilders by swallowing a glass full of raw eggs, but he failed to mention that raw eggs and the foods that contain them, such as egg nog, certain custards and tiramisu, are prime sources of the *salmonella* bacterium.

Another, of course, is raw or undercooked meat, the most dangerous being pork and poultry. Generations were raised on grey, overdone meat because of a fear of trichinosis, a parasitic disease caused by eating meat infected with the larvae of a specific type of roundworm. This condition has nearly always been associated with pork products; Thailand sees an annual spike in trichinosis cases around their astrological new year, when the eating of pork is traditional, and the World Health Organization reports that trichinosis is much more common in Eastern Europe, where pork is a much larger part of the diet and where the raising of livestock is much less regimented and much more household-oriented. But that should not lead you to believe that trichinosis doesn't happen in the good old U.S. of A. Though most commonly thought of as something you get from eating raw hotdogs (which is incorrect, as all hotdogs are pre-cooked before packaging ... though why anyone would want to eat them straight out of the package is beyond me), it can be contracted in the finest of kitchens if you're not too careful.

One of my patients was an ebullient woman and amazing cook named Rita DePasquale. Rita was the type of woman who lived life with both hands, which constantly moved as she talked about whichever topic moved her. She had seemingly boundless energy and was not shy about her kitchen skills, her husband John's belly providing some back-up to her claims. But she came in one day with her thirteen-year-old daughter in tow acting anything but her dynamic self. She was exhausted, she said, and her muscles ached, but she didn't feel like she had the flu. Her daughter claimed the exact same symptoms.

My first guess would have been mononucleosis, but Rita, in her late 30s by then, wasn't exactly a prime candidate. Then it occurred to me to ask them if they had eaten raw pork recently, because the symptoms pointed to possible trichinosis. They replied, "Of course we did," explaining that every time they made homemade sausages they tasted the combination of ground raw pork and seasonings before putting it into the casings. Fortunately for them, the diagnosis was made early and they were quickly treated and cured.

Raw pork is just one medium of transmission, and trichinosis just one illness. One of my patients contracted toxoplasmosis, a relatively benign parasitic infection that can nonetheless cause damage or death in certain individuals, by tasting raw hamburger for her meatball mixture; something to think about next time you order steak tartare. While in training over thirty years ago, my colleagues and I witnessed a completely unexpected outbreak of *Diphyllobothrium latum*, the longest tapeworm known to infect humans, among elderly Jewish housewives in the Bronx. The cause? While making gefilte fish, these women were tasting the mixture of ground raw fish to test for seasoning before cooking. Gefilte fish, a much loved delicacy fit only for the most discerning of epicures, is a mixture of carp, perch, pike, and whitefish, the last two being known carriers of *Diphyllobothrium latum*.

And, as if this business wasn't making you paranoid enough about the horrors lurking in your kitchen, there are methods of transmission of illness that don't even necessarily have to do with food itself. I'm sure that we're all familiar with the term "typhoid Mary," if only as something heard or read. But some of us may not be familiar with the story behind the name. "Typhoid Mary" was the disparaging name given to Mary Mallon, an Irish immigrant in the late 19th century who unwittingly carried and spread typhoid fever (itself caused by a type of *Salmonella* bacterium) as a cook and maid in early 20th century New York. As a healthy carrier of the disease, she infected people by passing the bacterium to the food she handled via her unwashed hands. So obviously sanitation and hygiene are also parts of the food poisoning equation. To bring the situation into perspective with a more modern tale, I once diagnosed two family members with hepatitis A after their visiting cousin inadvertently infected them during a family meal. As Asian immigrants, they had a habit of eating their meals "family style," picking their courses piece-by-piece with their chopsticks from a large community bowl, and it was through the chopsticks that the cousin had introduced the hepatitis virus into the serving bowl.

• • •

If you take precautions to wash your food and hands thoroughly, and cook your food completely, you should be able to avoid a majority of food-borne illness. And if you treat the symptoms promptly and seek appropriate medical attention, you will recover to dine again another day. As mentioned already, the majority of these illnesses can be prevented by conscientious preparation and cleaning around the kitchen, as well as cooking your meats fully (or at least on the outside for steak; see the following case file). If you're willing to make choices based more on common sense, logic, and basic health standards rather than cultural norms, rituals, or other internal and external pressures to behave a certain way, you'll be more likely to share good times with each other rather than contagious diseases. And if you follow this simple advice and pay prompt attention to any symptoms of food-related illness, you'll spend less time hugging the "porcelain god" and more time enjoying the life God gave you.

Food Poisoning—Signs & Prevention

SIGNS/SYMPTOMS OF GENERAL FOOD POISONING:

Depending on the type of food poisoning, symptoms can begin anywhere from a few hours to several days after eating contaminated food. The typical symptoms include abdominal pain, diarrhea, vomiting, and fever. Some forms of food poisoning will have vomiting without fever. And one of the most dangerous types, botulism, attacks the nervous system and exhibits signs of paralysis.

SIGNS / SYMPTOMS OF SPECIFIC FOOD POISONING:

- *Staphylococcus pre-formed toxins:* Symptoms start within the first 4 hours of a meal; be especially suspicious if the meal included ham, poultry, mayonnaise based salads, creamy pastries, fried rice, or vegetables.
- *Clostridium Perfringens:* Illness occurs 10 to 14 hours after a meal; be especially suspicious if the meal consisted of Mexican food, gravy, beef, or poultry.
- *Salmonella:* Symptoms typically include fever, abdominal cramps, diarrhea, headache, and sometimes vomiting, usually developing 12 to 72 hours after exposure to contaminated food. In those with poor underlying health or weak immune systems,

it can enter the bloodstream and cause infections, which can sometimes be life-threatening. These symptoms, along with loss of appetite, can last for several days. Dehydration, especially among infants, can be severe.

- *E. coli:* Symptoms often begin within 3 to 4 days, but can occur up to 8 days after becoming infected. *E. coli* is the cause of most traveler's diarrhea. Some people have no symptoms. Nevertheless, they can still pass the infection to others. Common signs and symptoms include diarrhea, abdominal cramping, nausea, dehydration, low-grade or no fever, and in extreme cases hemolytic uremic syndrome (HUS), a serious complication that can cause kidney failure, seizures, and even death. Because it can take eight days for symptoms to start, most patients get sick either on their return trip or when they get home. (That's one reason I never give antibiotics to travelers who are going away for that week's vacation.)
- *Shigella:* Symptoms of shigellosis typically begin a day or two after exposure to contaminated substance. One of the most common signs is diarrhea, often bloody. Other symptoms can include abdominal cramps and fever.
- *Trichinosis.* Symptoms can be mild (including nausea, diarrhea, vomiting, fatigue, fever, abdominal discomfort, itchy skin, and headache) to more severe (extreme versions of the above, as well as chills, eye swelling, aching joints and muscles, difficulty coordinating movement, and heart and breathing problems). The degree of severity can relate to the quantity of infectious worms consumed in the meat. Mild cases are often believed to be the flu or another common illness, and aren't diagnosed.

PRESCRIPTION
- General treatment of food poisoning, except botulism, deals mainly with preventing dehydration by putting back the fluids and electrolytes lost through vomiting and diarrhea. Dehydration is more common in young children, the elderly, and people taking diuretics. Drink plenty of Gatorade. In severe cases, a doctor can prescribe fluids intravenously.
- If the symptoms are severe, consult your doctor; he or she can prescribe medication to stop abdominal cramping and vomiting.

- If you feel you've contracted food poisoning it's a good idea to modify your diet. If you're suffering from vomiting or diarrhea don't eat, but drink only clear liquids, frequently but in small amounts. After the symptoms stop you might want to stick to a diet of bland, easy to digest foods for a few days. And drink lots of Gatorade.
- As mentioned earlier, take one *Saccharomyces boulardii* daily to prevent food poisoning and treat diarrhea.
- If difficulty speaking, swallowing, breathing, or other forms of paralysis occur, *seek immediate medical attention.*
- As previously stated, to prevent many of these maladies, wash your hands often, wash and cook your food thoroughly, and wash all utensils and food preparation areas completely.
- Make sure your refrigerator is cooler than 40 degrees F. Bacteria start multiplying at 40 degrees or more.
- Make sure your meats are cooked to a heat of 167 degrees F or more. That is the temperature that kills *Salmonella.*
- The family that shares a dinner plate together gets sick together. In other words, double dipping can be dangerous. Bottom line: if you share food in the Asian fashion, you are increasing your chances of sharing a lot more than you bargain for. My advice: it isn't worth the wok it came from!
- If you suspect you are suffering from any of these, keep well-hydrated and modify your diet to clear liquids and lots of preparations similar to Gatorade. If symptoms become severe or any form of paralysis occurs, *seek immediate medical attention.*
- While most of these illnesses will resolve on their own, it's always a safe practice to pay your health professional a visit.

PAY MORE ATTENTION TO YOUR COOKING HABITS!!!

- If you can avoid it, try not to taste-test raw meats. Instead, try cooking a small amount to test, and then prepare the rest.
- When handling raw meats, wash your hands before handling other foods to prevent transferring bacteria.
- Whether handling raw meat or not, be sure to wash your hands prior to food preparation and service (those signs in restaurant bathrooms are there for a reason).

- When at all possible, cook your meat thoroughly. Improperly cooked chicken and turkey are prime sources of "poultry salmonella." Steak can be served rare inside, as long as the outside was cooked. If one infected chicken is quartered and then mixed with other chicken parts, then all will be infected. If one steak is infected and is minced into chopped meat, then all of the chopped meat is contaminated. Hence the chicken and hamburger have to be cooked inside and not the steak. There has been a tendency for newer chefs to serve pork rare or pink. Based on what I've seen in my medical practice—and again, good old-fashioned common sense—I think that is a big mistake.
- Wash all produce thoroughly.

Prognosis

Food poisoning is a pretty common occurrence and rarely life threatening. If you take precautions to wash your food (and hands) thoroughly and cook your food completely, you should be able to avoid a majority of food-borne illness. And if you treat the symptoms promptly and seek appropriate medical attention, you will recover to dine again another day.

Don't Be Too Rash

Antibiotics are such a commonplace part of our lives that it is beginning to seem that we can't get away from them for even a minute, whether we're sick or not. They are not only in our medicine cabinets, but in our meat and our milk and other foods. On top of which, changes in the understanding of how certain conditions come to exist and affect the body—heart disease and some types of arthritis are two examples—have led to antibiotics being used in instances that would not have occurred to doctors only a decade ago. This has led some to fear the proliferation of this one-time "miracle drug" (and with some reason, I might add) and decry it in high profile ad and information campaigns. But before we start to think of the antibiotic class of drugs as a problem in and of itself, it's worthwhile to remember all the good they have done and can do.

It was just about a century ago that the very first antibiotic came into being. Arsphenamine, marketed under the name Salvarsan, was only effective against one specific class of bacteria. But that scientific class, the spirochete, is at the root of a surprising variety of illnesses and diseases: Weil's disease, relapsing fever (similar to typhus, but currently only deadly in 1% of cases that receive treatment), syphilis, each of which was quite serious in the days before effective treatments. Today, especially in the northeastern United States, we have been invaded by another spirochete-related disease: Lyme disease. Like other spirochetal infections, Lyme disease can lead to much more serious secondary and tertiary conditions that affect the musculoskeletal and nervous systems (among much else), and may lead to cardiac, neurological, psychiatric, and a host of other problems.

There are many similarities in the disease's presentation with syphilis, especially the varying types of rashes. We talk of the classic bull's-eye rash of Lyme disease, but the diagnosis of Lyme disease and related conditions is tricky. The infected tick that carries Lyme disease often also carries infections such as ehrlichiosis, babesiosis, and others not yet identified. On top of which, people may have varying symptoms or none at all. Signs and symptoms of the flu (weakness,

117

joint aches, fever) in the middle of the summertime, with or without a rash, are now considered to be indicative of Lyme disease until proven otherwise. Sometimes blinding, unexplainable headaches are a symptom of the acute (immediate or short-term) stage of Lyme disease; perhaps a precursor to the encephalitis that can be a manifestation of the chronic form of the disease later on. Lyme patients have shown up in emergency rooms with such severe headaches that some have claimed they considered shooting themselves rather than continue to suffer the pain.

• • •

Late one evening, I was called to our local emergency room to meet with Westchester County Executive Andrew Spano. Though probably not a nationally known name, Andy Spano is quite the newsworthy figure in my neck of the woods. As a Democratic executive officer of a traditionally Republican-leaning county with the eighth highest per capita income in the country, Spano has made a name for himself in lower New England and parts of the Mid-Atlantic region via his efforts at conservation and on behalf of lower-income residents of the county, as well as through his decision to recognize the validity of marriages of gay citizens so long as they were performed in a place where such ceremonies are legal (Belgium, Canada, The Netherlands, South Africa, Spain, and the state of Massachusetts), a decision he made on the very same day the U.S. Senate took its vote on the proposed constitutional amendment banning same-sex marriages.

Spano met me at the emergency room feeling feverish, weak, and exhausted. A preliminary screening test revealed low white blood cell and platelet counts, suggestive of tick-borne ehrlichiosis, but his more comprehensive blood tests were negative for all the commonly diagnosed tick diseases. By this time (the late 1990's) doctors across North America were quite familiar with Lyme disease, the mechanism of transmission by deer ticks having been positively identified a decade earlier, but we still thought to look for the "bull's eye" rash for confirmation. Despite the fact that I strongly suspected some kind of tick-borne infection, Spano presented without a rash or any type of skin disturbance. When asked, he responded that he had not been in any areas that day or even that week where he would have been likely to pick up a tick.

Lyme disease, like other spirochetal diseases and many infections in general, must be treated effectively in its acute stage to prevent it from taking root and progressing to chronic disease. The diagnosis has to be made on the first visit and can take up to three weeks to confirm in the laboratory. The common treatment is a course of doxycycline, a relatively powerful antibiotic that is also used to ward off malaria and is effective against the bacterium that causes bubonic plague. Because careless administration of antibiotics is a likely reason for the current prevalence of antibiotic-resistant infections like MRSA, it is best that doctors hold them in reserve if there's a reasonable amount of doubt as to what exactly is being treated. But I also knew the type of misery Lyme disease can cause in both the short and long run. Regardless of what his blood tests said, everything else pointed to Lyme, ehrlichiosis, or another tick-related infection. So I made sure he received treatment for these on that first visit to the E.R.

The tests were still negative the next week, as well as the week afterward. Three and one-half weeks after he had been in the emergency room, his tests finally turned positive. Further investigation revealed that Andy had inspected a county golf course the week before his visit to the emergency room. Although he could not identify a tick bite, he did recall that there had been a tiny scratch on his ankle.

His ordeal with the Lyme infection helped draw local attention to the disease, and the county then came forward with a public information campaign promoting behavior to avoid and reduce the incidences of infection (the wearing of high socks, use of insect repellents containing DEET, careful examination of the body for ticks after any time in the woods or high grass, etc.), which certainly had an impact.

• • •

There are two lessons (at least!) that we can learn from Andy Spano's experience with Lyme disease. The simplest one, but perhaps the more important, I'll discuss first:

Lyme Disease

SIGNS & SYMPTOMS OF LYME DISEASE:

- Flu-like symptoms (muscle aches, weakness and fatigue) during the summer in endemic areas is considered Lyme disease until proven otherwise. This may or may not be associated with fever. Especially significant is an associated severe headache.
- 60% of patients will have knowledge of a tick bite.
- 85% will have some type of bodily rash. Most of the time it will look like a bull's eye.
- The bull's eye rash may be multiple, all over the body, or just in one single spot. It is usually not at the site of the initial tick bite.
- If not treated, a few weeks after the initial infection one may develop Bell's palsy (weakness and usually transient paralysis of one side of the face).
- 2-6 months later, if still untreated, one may develop arthritis (usually in one large joint), carditis, or unusual neurologic symptoms.

PRESCRIPTION:

- An ounce of prevention is worth a pound of cure. Wearing socks and shoes and using repellent sprays are necessary in grassy areas.
- Once bitten, prevention of the disease can usually be accomplished by taking 200mg of doxycycline within 24 hours of the bite (there are other antibiotics available for those that have tetracycline allergy). Laboratory tests are then ordered three weeks later, unless symptoms of the disease occur.
- The disease is easily treated with three weeks of oral antibiotics.
- All patients with sudden joint swelling, Bell's palsy, cardiac abnormalities, or acute mental changes should be suspected of having Lyme and therefore be tested for the disease.
- Bell's palsy and mental changes require a spinal tap for the appropriate diagnosis of neurologic Lyme, as the therapy would have to be given intravenously. Because of the toxicity of IV antibiotics, the bacteria of Lyme or its antigens must be present in the spinal fluid for this kind of therapy. If the bacteria or its antigens are not present, there was no neurologic infection.

- In the case of Bell's palsy, the other known cause, the herpes simplex virus, is diagnosed by the use of blood tests.
- Arthritis due to Lyme is usually treated with oral antibiotics; if there is no improvement, IV antibiotics are then used.
- IV antibiotics are also used for cardiac manifestations of Lyme.

PROGNOSIS:

A cottage industry has grown in the Northeast, which often preys upon people who think they have Lyme disease but have not been diagnosed as such by mainstream physicians. Ninety percent of patients who are told they have manifestations of chronic Lyme actually have never had the disease to begin with. These patients are usually given three to four months (often up to twelve months) of intravenous antibiotic therapy (starting at $150 a shot), for a disease they never had.

Mainstream infectious disease experts and rheumatologists have strict guidelines for the use of IV antibiotics (for neurologic and cardiac Lyme and otherwise), and this is limited to three weeks, certainly not three months. I have never heard of a self proclaimed Lyme specialist who actually was a specialist in infectious disease. Many of these Lyme "specialists" are very wealthy, as their clientele's insurance pays out that $150-or-more daily IV rate. The sad part, in many cases, is that more serious illnesses go undiagnosed.

If you present with any of the above symptoms and you seek immediate medical attention, your chances of effectively dealing with the disease are high. If you are told that you have a chronic disease and need more then three weeks of an IV antibiotic, however, seek a second opinion by an infectious disease expert as well as a mainstream neurologist.

A delay in the treatment of any illness, particularly an infection, can lead to unwanted and deleterious consequences. Though not every single instance of an illness that is difficult to definitively diagnose is a health disaster waiting to happen, medical students are taught classic sets of symptoms of specific diseases and conditions for a reason: so that when they become licensed, practicing healers they can then practically apply that knowledge to the work of healing. Just as there are certain classic findings suggestive of Lyme and ehrlichiosis, so there are for any number of infirmities. But because doctors sometimes forget the fact that one could have negative tests for three weeks while still suffering from a real and definable disease, and because so many physicians in the United States live in mortal fear of knee-jerk lawsuits of advantage and convenience—as well as the ones with merit, which are a thousand times worse—the diseases and their unwanted consequences go undiagnosed and therefore untreated.

One of the most extreme examples of such a thing happening is the story surrounding the unfortunate death of Muppet creator Jim Henson. While at work one day in May of 1990, Henson began to feel ill with what he thought was a bad case of the flu. His physician suspected pneumonia; but an examination turned up no such evidence, so he sent Henson home with the classic prescribed treatment of aspirin and rest. The next day Henson was coughing up blood, and by the following day he was unable to breathe on his own. He was immediately admitted to New York Hospital, where he was found to have abscesses in his lungs. He was placed on a ventilator to help with his breathing, but he soon went into massive organ failure and died. The time from his initial examination to his death at the hospital was just over 72 hours, about four calendar days. Jim Henson was only 53 years old.

What Henson first thought was the flu, and what his doctor initially mistook for pneumonia, was actually a late-stage manifestation of *Streptococcus pyogenes,* a severe streptococcal infection. To this day no one knows the source of Henson's infection, but *S. pyogenes* usually gets its start in the throat or on the skin; in its milder forms it causes strep throat and impetigo. But in some cases an infection with *S. pyogenes* can lead to cellulitis (a skin infection that can spread to the underlying tissues, bloodstream, and lymphatic system), scarlet fever, and necrotizing fasciitis ("the flesh-eating disease"). In Jim Henson's case, though he was initially reported to have died of bacterial pneumonia, the doctor heading the team that treated Henson believed that he died of toxic shock syndrome caused by his infection. He also believed that if Henson had come to the hospital a few hours earlier, antibiotics could have saved his life.

As a much less deadly example, a mother once called me because she was at wit's end as to what to do about her daughter who was studying in Florence, Italy, for her third year of college. Unlike many of the stories in this book that involve Italy, I was contacted in this case not for my familiarity with *Italia* or *la bella lingua,* but because the girl had been seriously ill yet had not been diagnosed by the doctors that were tending to her in *Firenze*. She had been weak, exhausted, without appetite but with a high fever. All the proper blood tests were done the week before, but no diagnosis was made. Even after treatment with two different sets of antibiotics, the child continued to weaken and lose weight.

After explaining the situation to me, we telephoned the daughter together and I asked if she had lumps behind both ears. She did. There are only a small number of diseases in the world that cause bilateral post-auricular lymphadenopathy (swollen glands behind both ears); among them are mononucleosis, tuberculosis, and leishmaniasis. If it was tuberculosis, the girl would have presented with some sort of pulmonary symptom, most likely a phlegm-producing cough, along with her other symptoms. And it most likely wasn't leishmaniasis, which is caused by parasites transmitted through the bite of a sand fly, thereby earning it one of the more entertaining and—at the moment—sadly relevant casual names in medicine: Baghdad Boil. Proceeding from that assessment, oral cortisone was ordered, antibiotics being ineffective against mononucleosis because it is caused by a virus, and the daughter was said to be "ninety percent better" the next day. A miraculous turnaround. The mono test was repeated one week later and came back positive.

Each of these cases supports the approach that once the diagnosis is made clinically, treatment has to be initiated immediately, even in the face of initial negative blood tests. Most people contract things like strep and mono as children, and the symptoms are usually innocuous or non-existent. It is when childhood diseases are contracted as teens or young adults that the patients tend to get really sick.

A good case in point of the above, though on a massive scale, is the impact of chicken pox on teenage and adult Puerto Ricans. Up until the 1990s, chicken pox was not very prevalent in Puerto Rico, with fewer than 200 cases per 100,000 people as late as 1990. The virus somehow or another did not thrive in that climate. But with the increased mobility, heightened prosperity, and declining airfares of the last decade of the 20th century, Puerto Ricans were quickly introduced to the virus and many became deathly ill. This is because chicken pox, though usually minor and tolerable in children, is a much more active and severe condition in adults, potentially leading to all sorts of nasty complications down the road (pneumonia and encephalitis in the shorter term, and the painful condition known as shingles later in life). In fact, though there are usually 100 or fewer deaths from chicken pox each year in the United States, 80% of those who do die from the disease are aged 20 or over. In the cases of Puerto Ricans first contracting chicken pox, it wasn't uncommon for adults to die from varicella pneumonia as an immediate complication. Nowadays, though, varicella protective vaccine has reduced deaths tremendously, and Puerto Ricans given the varicella vaccine as young-sters in Puerto Rico developed the same immunity as mainlanders.

• • •

There is a second lesson to be learned from Andrew Spano's Lyme dis-ease experience, and it carries through some of the other cases we've discussed here and elsewhere. That lesson is about the sometimes unfortunate, sometimes maddening, sometimes beneficial, but near-ly always curious intersection of illness, fame, politics, and (some-times, if enough is at stake) business.

Political leaders and celebrities who are stricken by an illness, either directly or by its proximity to their lives, are usually the spearheads in paving the way for education, funding, research, or other progress in the battle against that same illness. Franklin Delano Roosevelt spent much of his inheritance in setting up a treatment center for the post effects of polio, the disease that left him paralyzed for the last twenty-four years of his life.[9] The actor Christopher Reeve and his wife did exhaustive work on behalf of those suffering from spinal cord injuries and physical disabilities after Reeve himself was paralyzed from the neck down after a horse riding accident, setting up research and treat-ment institutes and advocating before the government for greater funding and fewer restrictions on relevant research. New York State Senator Vincent Leibell, moved by the suffering of personal friends dying of cancer, is asking the state senate to legalize the medical use of marijuana. Certainly a bold and courageous move for any politician, but more so for a high-ranking Republican, which he happens to be.

Sometimes these people will even go the extra mile and put them-selves at considerable risk to do their advocacy work. Earvin "Magic" Johnson and Elizabeth Glaser, wife of *Starsky & Hutch* actor Paul

---

9   Modern medical science points to Roosevelt having suffered from Guillain–Barre syndrome rather than polio, but why let that get in the way of a good story?

Michael Glaser, did much to change the public perception of AIDS at a time when general misconceptions and ignorance about the disease frequently led to acts of cruelty and violence against sufferers. Another case in point involves our old friend Andy Spano.

Just after the terrorist attacks of Sept. 11, 2001, New York State rushed to set up a health &treatment program for first-responders. Many of the state's individual counties followed suit, Westchester County in particular because of its proximity to New York City. The horrible shock of that day was aggravated further by the talk that had been swirling through the media for the past decade about the weapons potentially at the disposal of both our real and imagined enemies: portable nuclear devices, nerve agents, biological weapons. After the anthrax episodes that followed on the heels of the September 11 attacks, greater attention began to be paid to the threat of biological attack. There was a near-immediate consensus in the halls of power that smallpox was a more likely agent to fear than anthrax due to its more grandly lethal qualities, so part of the program was for first-responders to receive the smallpox vaccine.

Mandatory vaccination of schoolchildren against smallpox was discontinued in the United States in 1972, the disease considered eradicated here since 1949. The white, starburst shaped vaccination scar now serves as a sort of generational marker. At age 17, when I was a U.S. Navy (and subsequently a U.S. Marine) hospital corpsman, all military personnel received a smallpox vaccination upon induction and every four years thereafter. That is unless, as so often happens in the armed services, your records were lost or went missing. Then you received an extra series of shots (that fear of receiving extra shots was a good reason why corpsmen were treated with a lot of respect).

Considering the fact that generations of Americans had been safely vaccinated against smallpox, there was a surprising amount of negativity regarding the safety of the vaccine. To show that there was no harm, Spano, in front of the press corps, took a smallpox vaccination. Applause was offered and backs were patted, and that appeared to be the end of it. But when Spano came to me six months later for his annual physical, I found his vaccination site still festering as if he had just been vaccinated only a few days before. Ordinarily the site festers for up to a week, after which a scab forms which itself falls off after a week or so, leaving the distinctive scar. This was, to put it mildly, out of the ordinary.

I immediately contacted the Centers for Disease Control in Atlanta. Unbeknownst to me, the primary physician, Spano had been the topic of great discussion amongst the specialists at the CDC. No one there had any experience with giving the vaccine over the previous thirty years, and each person I talked to was utterly baffled. Spano's case exhibited the longest festering site they had on record, and they were concerned that the disease could be developing right before them.

I remembered then that when we gave vaccinations in the military, the standard procedure was to keep the site of injection covered for three or four days to prevent person-to-person transmission, especially to people who weren't allowed to receive smallpox vaccine, such as those with severe dermatitis. In Spano's case, the Westchester County Health Department, under the CDC's guidelines, recommended Band-Aid coverage until the scab dried. They thought that keeping the wound covered continually was the proper care of the vaccine site. Instead, keeping it dry after three days was the way we took care of it in the late 1950s. So after telling the CDC of my decision, I removed the bandage from his arm and we waited.

Spano's injection site cleared up in two or three days after the Band-Aid was removed. Considering his age, he was probably as used to the idea of smallpox vaccination as I was. Though he could not have expected things to progress as they did, he never lost his head and performed a huge service to the public by proving that it is truly safe to take a smallpox vaccination.

• • •

All of the above examples are unquestionably good things. But sometimes the political climate surrounding a particular illness or related issue causes an opportunistic politician—or drug company—to take actions that range from the ineffective to the unethical. During the mid-1970s, because of the panic that ensued following the first few cases of Legionnaires disease in New York City, then-mayor Abe Beame ordered large tanker trucks with spray attachments to ride through the streets of the city, spraying water and washing the streets, showing the public that something was being done. Too bad that the causative bacteria for Legionnaires disease are found in water towers and large, roof-mounted air conditioning units. The message he tried to send was clear: the city was washing away germs. That message, however, was far from the truth. Approaching a public health issue from another angle, nearly all of America was at one time familiar with New York State's draconian Rockefeller drug laws, passed by Governor Nelson Rockefeller in 1973. In retrospect, it is difficult to say if the laws were an honest attempt to stem the rising health problem of narcotics addiction and abuse, a problem that only got worse over the thirty-two years that these laws were on the books, or just a sop to the voting public in an effort to convince them that something was being done. Either way, all the laws did was to fill up New York's prisons with countless non-violent, mostly minority offenders, where they soon learned to graduate to greater levels of crime and violence.

But it seems that we've almost come to expect this type of maneuvering from our elected officials. It's almost as if, when assessing their potential legacies, we judge our politicians on a sliding scale of severity of transgressions. For some reason, we usually seem much more outraged when we catch drug companies engaging in cold hearted business– and image-oriented trickery.

As I said much earlier, there are many drugs and remedies from past eras, as well as from the folk pharmacopoeia, that worked just fine but were replaced by drugs that were simply newer and more expensive, distinct advantages for the pharmaceutical companies. Often these drugs are much more toxic than the treatments they purport to replace, as they have to be taken orally to be distributed through the bloodstream rather than be directed to the source of the problem. Over the course of my career, I have seen many examples of this pharmaceutical greed.

As a military corpsman years ago, I came across many remedies that cost mere pennies per dosage yet were amazingly effective. Potassium permanganate is a mineral salt that has been used to remove excess iron from well water; but when its crystals are put in a bucket of water and dissolved it could and did cure the worst cases of athlete's foot after only two days of treatment. Its only "side effect," if it can even be so called, is that it temporarily stains the skin purple. Compare this to newer products like Lamisil, which take between a week and a month to remedy the problem and cost approximately $20.00 for a full course of treatment. Modern pharmaceutical houses have bought up the world's supply of potassium permanganate and kept it off the market, as if the fortunes of a company like Novartis Pharmaceuticals (perhaps better known by their earlier name,

Sandoz, and the makers of Lamisil) were based solely, or even primarily, on an athlete's foot remedy. Gentian violet, another inexpensive antifungal preparation, could have met the same fate if it were not a vital bacterial identification tool in medical laboratories (part of the gram stain method of identifying bacteria). Today, those who know it at all outside of the scientific community usually associate it, incorrectly, with the old-fashioned C. Howard's violet mints.

Once upon a time, the scrub soap "pHisoHex" was used in nearly every hospital in the country because of its ability to kill bacteria thanks to the active ingredient, hexachlorophene; the fact that it was incredibly cheap only sweetened its appeal. Patients with furunculosis (tender, pus-filled lumps caused by an inflammation of the hair follicles), pustular acne, and recurrent *Staph* infections would improve and often completely recover from their symptoms after two weeks of a regimen of pHisoHex showers twice a day. It was removed from general usage after publication of a report designating it a suspected carcinogen. The study that furnished the results in the report used gallons of hexachlorophene on lab mice; if one were to use the same experimental formula on humans, it would take tons of hexachlorophene to reproduce the same effect. Though it was later determined not to cause cancer, it is now only available by prescription.

On a related note, it seems the lion's share of the world quinine supply—used to treat leg cramps and malaria for just a few dollars per dosage, as well as the vital ingredient in tonic water—has just been bought up by a pharmaceutical house. Chronic charley horse sufferers and lovers of summertime cocktails, take note. With the quinine supply now privately owned, those same treatments will cost $100 dollars and more.

Sometimes a company or other entity will buy up the supply of a drug or drug component not necessarily to keep it off the market, but to make sure that there is only one source for it, giving that entity control over the market price of that substance. This is exactly how Armand Hammer (the oil tycoon, of course, not the baking soda) made not one, but two fortunes. First, he bought the world futures supply of coca leaf, used in producing an early recipe of Coca-Cola as well as in some pharmaceuticals. This insured that the Coca-Cola Company would have to purchase their supplies from him. Later, while working exporting pharmaceuticals, he noted that ginger was being used in an increasing number of new medicines as well as in a new soft drink—ginger ale, developed to soothe palates left dry by prohibition. Hammer promptly set about buying up the world futures supply of ginger.

Then there are times when demand is either artificially manipulated or actively encouraged by playing on insecurities or outright fear rather than need and purpose. This is an old, perhaps ancient tactic that can be traced back at least as far as the snake-oil salesmen from the travelling "medicine shows" of two centuries ago. But it has taken on new life with each passing era of history, as companies discovered that by capitalizing on garden variety situations they could push their wares, even develop new ones, to meet an "urgent need" that only their advertising campaigns had created. Thus did the makers of Sal Hepatica, a popular laxative in the early 20th century, create fear in the American heart of succumbing to "auto-intoxication," a condition that, so their advertisements led the consumer to believe, was the natural and inevitable outcome of episodic constipation.

A more recent example also hearkens back to those dark days of September 2001. After the anthrax scares that followed the attacks on New York and Washington, a new term entered the general lexicon, if only for a while: "Cipro," Bayer Pharmaceuticals' brand name for the synthetic antibiotic ciprofloxacin. Though Bayer was obviously not behind the episode, it could not have come at a better time for them. Facing the imminent expiration of their patent rights to Cipro, they were almost assured of losing their market share to generics when Cipro was touted as the only remedy to, or best drug for prevention of, inhalation anthrax. Bayer did nothing to discourage this idea, and took the opportunity to develop a new formulation (once-daily dosing, as opposed to the original twice-daily), thereby securing an extension of its original patent. It is now believed that the "mass deployment" of Cipro in the post-9/11 panic was a significant factor in the genesis and spread of bacteria that are highly resistant to antibiotics.[10]

Not only is this a timely example to illustrate my point, it brings this story full circle to the point I made at its opening, thank you very much.

---

[10] In addition to being made widely available in the wake of 9/11, ciprofloxacin and other antibiotics of its class have been added to livestock feed with increasing and alarming frequency.

Don't Forget to Breathe

THERE'S AN OLD SAYING that whoever is the calmest in a fire will be the one to find the door out.

Of course, this is no mean feat. Being calm during emergencies takes years and years of training. Training for any emergency involves clearing your mind of feeling to be able focus on the problem at hand and solve it, rather than dwelling on the potential for negative consequences that cloud the mind with panic, fear, and a helpless feeling of ... well, helplessness. It requires relaxing, calming, and dumping of all emotions; it also has a lot to do with concentrating on your breathing. Exclude all other thoughts and concentrate on your breathing. Breathing is the essence of life in many more ways than the obvious.

Controlling your breathing controls your mind and your body. Training in the martial arts, a hobby of mine, teaches a most unnatural way of breathing. It comes from the lower abdomen, with long inhaling and even longer exhalation. It takes an awful lot of practice, but helps replace the panting and blowing and coughing that an average person would experience if they had to run up a couple of flights of stairs or who experience an anxiety attack. Liken it to a cat suddenly threatened. It quickly arches its back and starts to take long, deep breaths, slowly inhaling and then exhaling with a long, slow hiss. The cat is preparing for an emergency by controlling the one thing that will keep it going—its breathing. The next components in dealing with emergencies are training and repetition. With proper breathing and a calm mind, the lessons learned through constant repetition kick in.

At age 17, as a corpsman in the navy stationed at Floyd Bennett Field in Brooklyn, we continuously trained for crashes. The night "my" first crash occurred, there were only two of us on duty. I got panicky as we drove our "meat wagon" onto the runway, thinking what we could do if there were thirty or forty seriously injured military souls on board? How could just the two of us do anything? Artie Schultz was my corpsman companion that fateful evening, and he said something I'll never forget: "Don't worry, just take care of one at a time. The seriously wounded first." Of course, memorable or not, that didn't alleviate my anxieties at the time. But the approach to the crash site did.

It turned out to be a private Cessna with just the pilot on board. The fire department arrived a few seconds before us and had gotten the bloodied pilot out of the wreckage and onto the tarmac. We ran up to the victim and Artie did something else I would never forget. He knelt down and started taking the pilot's pulse. As he did that, he looked all around, surveying the crash site.

The pulse taking was really just a subterfuge; the proverbial cat arching his back and hissing a breath. Artie really wasn't taking a pulse, he was using the technique to calm himself—breathe control and get control. Then he jumped into action. He had been developing a plan of action all along. Years later, as the ambulance attendant for Long Island Jewish Hospital, I practiced the same "pulse taking" technique to get my own emotions under control and assess each situation personally and individually. Whether it was a car crash or a building fire, I used this technique to develop a sense of calm under fire. Now there is an automatic reflex that kicks in during an emergency—whether it's while flying my plane or taking care of critically ill patients, I stay calm.

If you panic in a crisis, you are likely to lose the battle before you even begin the fight. But the presence of mind that can save lives is always just a deep breath and pulse beat away. In a more practical sense, dealing with emergencies requires preparation by LAP:

1. Learn everything about the problem,

2. Apply your knowledge by studying, and

3. Practice, Practice, Practice.

Policemen, firemen, soldiers, EMTs, airline pilots, teachers, all of them continually practice their skills and train for emergencies. Developing and practicing your skills for emergencies will make you safer, confident, and competent.

Of course, the "P" also stands for Preparation. If you are concerned that you won't know what to do in a crisis, large or small, there is no time like the present to begin to change that. Think about the emergencies that you could potentially face. Be realistic and honest. Then make a list of how to deal with them. Take a course in basic first aid and C.P.R.; learn how to treat bleeding, burns, choking, and poisoning; learn how to put out small household fires before they become huge house fires, and make sure you have a fire extinguisher charged and ready for the job; know where your water shut-off valve and your electric master switch are.

Experience may be the best teacher, but it's probably better to hear these lessons from a former student rather than learn them directly from the instructor.

Crisis Prep

SIGNS & SYMPTOMS YOU MAY NOT BE ABLE TO HOLD IT TOGETHER IN A CRISIS

- You are concerned that you won't know what to do if something happens.
- You have never thought of emergency planning.
- You don't know if you have a fire extinguisher or where it might be.
- You don't know the location of your water supply shut-off valve or your electrical system's master switch.
- You don't know any first aid or haven't studied it since high school.

PRESCRIPTION

- Make a list of the most common emergencies you will encounter, and then make a plan to deal with them.
- Learn CPR and first aid, if only for the sake of your loved ones. Take a course at the American Red Cross or one sponsored by the American Heart Association. You can even take one online.
- At minimum, learn what to do for poisoning, choking, bleeding, and burns. That is, learn to do your ABCs:
  1. is the Airway clear?
  2. is the patient Breathing (and is their breathing absent, labored, or normal)?
  3. is the Circulation flowing? (i.e., check the tone of the victim's skin for flush, pallor, or other abnormalities)
- Everyone working in a hospital learns mnemonics for fire control and how to put them into effect. RACE stands for Rescue

someone who is trapped, Alarm to be sounded, Contain or control the area, and Extinguish the fire.

- PASS applies to the use of a fire extinguisher: Pull the pin, Aim the extinguisher, Squeeze the handle, and Spray the area.
- Learn how to make and use mnemonics for any situation you deem important. Though you may laugh at the simplicity of the device, it is an excellent tool to help memorize important things.
- Know where your circuit breaker is, remembering that electrical fires require that the electricity be turned off for that particular appliance (pull out the plug and turn off the circuit breaker).
- Take the time to label all the shut off valves associated with your faucets, showers, commodes, sinks, etc. When I purchased my first home, I discovered a leaking pipe in the boiler room. I tried putting towels around the pipe and called for help. My next door neighbor entered, surveyed the scene for a second, then reached over and closed a valve right next to my nose, which controlled the water flow in the leaking valve. Embarrassing, but informative.
- Have fire extinguishers placed in rooms that have heavy equipment and place fire detectors in appropriate places. Every year on your birthday, check the extinguishers and change the detectors' batteries.

Eat Less, Lose Weight

A QUICK LOSS OR GAIN of five pounds can make a physician suspicious.

Estelle was looking great and I asked her what kind of diet she was on. "Doc," she said, "you told me to lose thirty pounds and I lost thirty-five." She said she wasn't on any diet. Weight loss may be fashionable as well as desirable, but if it is occurring without being on a diet or fitness regimen, something might be wrong. Estelle had something wrong. Fortunately, it was a controlled form of diabetes.

Illness and medication aside, people gain weight from eating more calories that they can burn off. Eat and drink too many calories and you become fat. The simple formula for understanding weight and weight gain or loss is: eleven times your body weight. If you weigh 150 pounds, you multiply 11 x 150; this will give you the number of calories needed to maintain your present body weight. A 150-pound person requires 1,650 calories as a daily intake to sustain their current weight. If that 150-pound person eats more than 1,650 calories in one day, they will gain weight. If they eat less than 1,650 calories, they will lose weight. If they ate 500 calories less a day, at the end of one week their body would have to burn off 3,500 calories of fat or protein to make up the required deficit (500 x 7 days). Every 3,500-calorie loss will equal a one-pound loss. Deducting more than 500 calories a day will help you lose more quickly. To prevent loss of muscle while on a diet, one must make sure they eat at least 300 calories of protein daily. When deprived of calories, muscle as well as fat will lose mass. We want to preserve muscle at the expense of fat.

The body is like a bank account; it knows how much you put in and how much you take out. Every diet works by this principle. You can't lose weight if you eat too many calories per day. Call it Atkins, Doctor's Fast, South Beach, or the Zone: they all wind up keeping you eating a lower caloric intake than eleven times your body weight per day.

Exercise is also important not just for weight loss, but for toning and increasing one's basic metabolism. It gets your body's system working faster and more efficiently. Your heart pumps more efficiently, your cardiac output is better, and your body disposes more easily of cellular waste and byproducts. You feel much better about yourself and your body as you go from flabby to toned to muscled.

But what type of exercise to pursue?

Well, jogging one mile burns off 100 calories. Walking one mile burns off the same 100 calories, just more slowly. In order to lose one pound you would have to burn off 3,500 calories. That is, you would have to jog thirty-five miles. Most of us can't jog thirty-five miles a week, let alone in one day. But if we did manage such a feat, there goes a pound a week. The average person can begin jogging a half-mile a day and each week add an additional quarter of a mile. After eight weeks, a two-mile day is a great way to help rev up our metabolism. It also burns that extra 200 calories a day. That's not much, but it would allow you to cheat and eat a couple of Oreo cookies or a very small serving of chocolate gelato when you finally get to your goal weight.

The long-term goal is to learn what calories are, where they come from and how to manage them. The purpose is to live a healthy life as well as a happy one. Weight loss isn't something we just will to happen, it has to be associated with active participation by eating fewer calories on purpose. If you are losing weight without trying or have lost your appetite, it's time to see your doctor.

Nutritional Info Table

There are many ways that you can take an active roll in disease prevention. One excellent way to be proactive is to be aware of what exactly it is that you are putting into your body. Below is a comparison list of food: some good, some bad. And even though some of the most unhealthful foods taste oh-so-good, or claim to be better for you than they actually are, don't be fooled. You must read labels and know what you are consuming.

- **Pepperidge Farm Original Flaky Crust Roasted Chicken Pot Pie:** A.K.A, "artery crust." This has 1,000 calories and 31 grams of artery clogging fat.
- **McDonald's Chicken Selects Premium Breast Strips:** Though you may assume chicken is inherently healthier than any burger, this fast-food treat is in fact quite a "strip tease." A five strip order has 630 calories and 11 grams of fat.

- The Cheesecake Factory's Original and 6-Carb Cheesecake has 610 calories per slice, with 29 grams of saturated fat (that's 1½ days' supply).
- Ben & Jerry's, Haagen-Dazs, and Dove ice cream each squeeze 300 calories and 13 grams of saturated fat (that's half a days worth) into a ½ cup.
- A single Mrs. Fields milk chocolate & walnuts cookie has 300 calories, 50 grams of fat, and 6 teaspoons of sugar.
- They call it coffee but it's really a milk shake: a Starbucks Venti Strawberries & Frappuccino Blended Crème with whipped cream contains 770 calories and 19 grams of fat.
- A Burger King king-size order of french fries has 600 calories, as well as ¾ of your USDA maximum recommended daily allowance of fat.
- A half can of Campbell's red and white label condensed soups serves up more than half a person's daily quota of salt.
- Hershey crams 200 calories, 8 grams of saturated fat, and more than 4 teaspoons of sugar into each six-count pack of their Swoops candy.
- A Mint Chip Dazzler at Haagen-Dazs stores has 1,270 calories and 38 grams of saturated fat.
- Containered or frozen fruit juices such as orange or apple have four times the amount of sugar and calories as the same amount of a whole fruit or freshly squeezed juice.
- Most breakfast cereals contain tons of sugar, corn syrup, starch, and processed, unhealthy ingredients.

ON THE OTHER HAND …

- Sweet potatoes, a nutritional all-star, are loaded with carotinoids (which devour free radicals and therefore may lower your risk of certain cancers), vitamin C, potassium, and fiber.
- Grape tomatoes are sweeter and firmer than other tomatoes, and their bite-size shape makes them perfect for snacking, dipping, or salads. They are loaded with vitamins C and A, and they deliver both fiber and flavor.
- FOR WOMEN ONLY—Fat-free and 1% milk are excellent sources of calcium, vitamins and protein, with no artery clogging fat. (Recent data show a potential link between some types of low-fat and fat-free milk and prostate cancer in men).

- **Blueberries** are rich in fiber, vitamin C, and antioxidants, as well as absolutely delicious. I have a healthy Russian émigré patient who eats two cartons every day!
- The omega-3 fats in **fatty fresh fish** like wild salmon can help reduce the risk of sudden, fatal heart attacks.
- **Whole grain rye crackers** like Wasa, Ry Krisp and Ryvita—usually called "crispbreads"—are loaded with fiber and are usually fat free.
- Try regular or "quick cooking" **whole grain brown rice** instead of enriched white rice. This way you don't lose the fiber, magnesium, vitamins E and B6, copper, and zinc that are "enriched" out of white rice.
- A growing number of food stores sell peeled, seeded, cut, and ready to go bags of diced **butternut squash**. Every half cup has 5 grams of fiber and loads of vitamins A and C.
- **Greens like kale, spinach, and broccoli** are nutritional gems. They are loaded with vitamin C, carotenoids, calcium, folate, potassium, and fiber.
- An **apple** every day, or even an orange, really will keep the doctor away. Note, however, that the saying never mentioned pre-packaged juices.
- The fattening of America is partly due to breakfast cereals. Instead of all that sugar, try **Kashi** cereals, which are made with healthy ingredients.

Remember: You are what you eat and you must be responsible for what you put inside of your body. Reduce your total fat intake by one half. Reduce your cholesterol consumption. Reduce your saturated fat intake. Reduce your over all consumption of sugar and sweets. Increase your consumption of fiber, grains, greens, and proteins. By reading labels and avoiding the above-mentioned foods, you can lower your risk of heart disease and many cancers.

All You Wanted to Know
About the Common Cold
But Were Too Hoarse to Ask

SOMETIMES PERCEPTION IS the same as the truth. Case in point: the most common ailment that brings people to physicians is the common cold, often associated with a sore throat.

Colds are caused by viruses and are self-limiting, usually lasting a week or less. If the symptoms last longer than a week, it probably is not a cold. People with sniffles, running noses and watery head congestion who have symptoms more then a week are probably suffering with allergies. Most sore throats are also due to viruses, but there is also the chance that strep bacterium is the cause. Children are prone to strep throats, and adults who have young children or who interact closely with young children (childcare providers, teachers, etc.) are usually the only adults who are prone to strep throats. But in other adults strep is extremely rare.

There is no way one can look inside a patient's throat and know whether it's a virus or strep throat, so cultures must be taken to determine whether strep is present or not. And though the instant strep culture is ninety-five percent accurate, there are many groups and types of strep that normally grow in our throats. Most need no antibiotic therapy. In fact, antibiotics are not used for any throat infection other then beta hemolytic, group A strep. They are not used for viruses, *Staph* or any other bacteria, including all other strep groups. Patients with group A, beta hemolytic infections all get symptomatically better on their own, even without antibiotics.

When they are used, antibiotics are given to prevent rheumatic fever. When we are infected with this type of strep, our bodies produce antibodies. These antibodies can cause damage to our own hearts if antibiotics are not given in a timely fashion, and this is the cause of rheumatic fever. Therefore antibiotics are given to prevent later complications and not to cure the sore throat. After twenty-four hours on antibiotics, the patient is no longer contagious.

But as I said, most sore throats are caused by a virus and easy to treat, like the common cold with which they are associated. There are other, even more benign (relatively benign, anyway) causes of a garden variety sore throat. Drinkers, smokers, and singers can develop muscle strain of the larynx and throat, causing sore throats. Outdoor and indoor pollutants and allergens make some susceptible to throat irritation, which will clear up once the irritant has been removed. People that awaken with a severe sore throat probably have clogged noses or sinuses, forcing them to breathe through their mouths as they sleep; this causes the driest and sorest throat ever. And acid reflux during the evening can irritate the throat and lungs, causing chronic sore throats and chronic coughing. And as it happens, I touch upon that in the very next chapter.

Common Cold Symptoms & Treatment

SIGNS AND SYMPTOMS THAT YOU MAY HAVE MORE THAN A COMMON COLD

- Severe and prolonged sore throat
- Difficulty breathing, swallowing or opening your mouth
- Joint pain
- Earache or fever over 101 degrees F
- Hoarseness that lasts more then two weeks
- Blood in saliva or phlegm
- Lumps in the neck

PRESCRIPTION

- Any drug allergy can cause sore throats; but if associated with a blistering rash, a doctor should be seen immediately.
- Mononucleosis is associated with swollen tonsils and swollen glands (especially behind the ears), as well as fatigue. This requires treatment with cortisone—never, ever take amoxicillin or ampicillin when you have mono, otherwise a terrible rash will ensue.
- Drug or alcohol abusers, smokers, and singers can develop muscle strain of the larynx and throat, causing sore throats; obviously discontinuance of bad habits is important.
- Outdoor pollutants as well as indoor pollutants (dog, cat, or bird

dander, or cigarette smoke), should be eliminated for those with susceptible allergies.
- Many virus infections (measles, chicken pox, croup), as well as bacterial infections (strep, dyptheria), are associated with sore throats.

Viral infections require no antibiotics, but certain strep and certainly dyptheria infections do.
- GERD (gastroesophageal reflux disease) causes acid reflux during the evening which can irritate the throat and lungs, causing chronic sore throats and chronic coughing. Elevate the head of your bed just two inches and take an antacid prior to sleep.
- Special attention should be given to those who have swallowing disorders or neck swelling; cancers of the tongue, throat, and larynx can cause sore throats and much worse (they're more common in smokers, drinkers, and singers).

PROGNOSIS

It's important to be aware of the signals our body sends us. Most of the time, a sore throat is a sore throat, due to a virus infection or a sinus inflammation. However, following the above guidelines will keep you and your Doctor on "speaking" terms.

Pneumonia 101

AND WHEN IS A COUGH MORE than just a cough? When your body, and your doctor, tell you so! Okay, perhaps this is not so venerably jokey. But the cough, a simple reflex contraction of the thoracic cavity to expel something irritating the throat or lungs, is one of the most misunderstood and misdiagnosed (by the layman, anyway) symptoms on the books.

Coughing is considered indicative of many illnesses and conditions—inherent lung diseases (chronic obstructive pulmonary disease or COPD, asthma, etc.) or post nasal drips or allergies. Sometimes a chronic cough can be caused by gastroesophageal reflux disease (GERD), or acid reflux. When lying down at night, gastric acid rises through the esophagus, leaking into the bronchial tree and causing, you guessed it: coughing. Taking antacids at night and elevating the head of the bed will prevent this common but less known cause of chronic coughing. Occasionally, people visiting certain parts of California (the San Joaquin Valley), as well as parts of Texas, Utah, Nevada, and New Mexico, develop a chronic cough due to a fungus, which oftentimes gets stirred up when there are heavy winds in these desert areas. Aptly named the San Joaquin Valley Fever, this fungal infection causes a cough, sometimes for months, which usually does not require treatment.

There are other ailments of which a chronic cough is considered emblematic. Tuberculosis, of course, though the average American is unlikely to encounter this outside of prisons or other densely populated institutional settings. Perhaps the most feared sickness, for both young and old, associated with a cough is pneumonia. Can't you just

143

hear your mother yelling to you across the years as you go out to "wear your hat, or you'll catch your death from pneumonia!!"

Despite its association with freezing weather or wet clothes, pneumonia is not uncommon even in sunny climes or dry areas. Many people, in fact, have something known as "walking pneumonia." This is a condition where the patient usually doesn't have a cough, but does have fever and, sometimes, associated upper respiratory symptoms such as a sore throat or head congestion. The diagnosis of walking pneumonia is usually made when the patient goes to see his or her doctor to get some sort of prescription for what they assume is a case of the flu or a cold or random virus. When the doctor listens to the chest of such patients, or looks at the X-ray ordered after hearing the odd crackling sounds the lungs make during this illness, pneumonia is found, much to the patient's surprise. For this reason, patients with a fever of unknown origin (i.e., with no localizing symptoms or findings) should have a chest X-ray to rule out walking pneumonia.

Most pneumonias, like most sore throats, are due to viruses and don't respond to antibiotics (to which only bacterial infections respond).[11] Like most viral infections, viral pneumonia is a gradually progressive disease: patients have malaise, weakness, and gradually develop cold symptoms and a cough. These symptoms may or may not be associated with fever and usually do not have greenish phlegm. Patients with influenza, especially young children and the elderly, can develop influenza pneumonia, which can be quite serious. Again, no antibiotics are indicated because this is a viral infection.

Bacterial pneumonias, on the other hand, start off abruptly. One is healthy one day and the next has sudden chills, which usually denote the onset of bacteria introduced into the bloodstream. After approximately two hours, the body responds with a fever and a cough that seems to come out of the blue (or the green, considering the amount of phlegm produced in these cases). The more shaking the chills produce, the higher the fever and more serious will be the infection. Patients with symptoms of bacterial pneumonias with very elevated white blood counts may have to be admitted to the hospital for intra-

---

11   There is a special class of organisms, known as Mycoplasma, that are neither virus nor bacteria and that also cause a type of pneumonia. These Mycoplasma also respond to some types of antibiotics.

venous therapy. However, if their fever isn't too high and their breathing capacity is not compromised, or there is no other significant underlying illness, they may be treated from home

Like most acute infections in other parts of the body, all forms of pneumonia, bacterial, viral, or atypical, should be diagnosed and treated in an urgent manner. Delay in identification may lead to the wrong treatment and, as a result, complications. But if one has no underlying disease (diabetes, COPD) and is not on one end of the age curve (child or the elderly), they can usually be successfully treated at home.

Pneumonia

SIGNS AND SYMPTOMS THAT YOUR COUGH MAY BE MORE THAN JUST A COUGH

- Like most viral infections, viral pneumonia is a gradually progressive disease. Patients have malaise, weakness, and gradually develop cold symptoms and a cough.
- These symptoms may or may not be associated with fever and usually do not have greenish phlegm.
- Bacterial pneumonias, on the other hand, start off abruptly. One is healthy one day and the next has sudden chills, fever, and a productive (greenish phlegm) cough. The cough comes "out of the blue," or "green" in this case.
- Patients with influenza can develop influenza pneumonia. They are sick with the flu and progressively get worse and worse, over the next 5-7 days. No antibiotics are indicated because this is a viral infection.
- This is in contradiction with patients who are suffering with the flu who are gradually improving. Suddenly, 4-7 days later, they develop chills, a new fever, and a productive cough. This is bacterial superinfection on top of a viral infection (the flu), and does require treatment with antibiotics.

PRESCRIPTION

- Patients with fever of unknown origin (no localizing symptoms or findings) should have a chest X-ray to rule out walking pneumonia.

- Patients with viral-like symptoms (gradual onset) almost never need antibiotics. During certain months and depending on geographic location, some virus-like pneumonias actually are due to mycoplasma infections. These infections do require antibiotic therapy.
- Patients with symptoms of bacterial pneumonias with very elevated white blood counts may have to be admitted to the hospital for intravenous therapy. However, if their fever isn't too high and their breathing capacity is not compromised, or if there is no other significant underlying illness, they may be treated from home.
- Usually a gram stain should be done on "deep seated" sputum to identify the specific bacteria (which will often be engulfed by the body's white blood cells).

Needed: Prescription for Apathy ... STAT!

CONTRARY TO POPULAR OPINION, hospitals and physicians offices aren't the safe havens one would think they are. When I was a medical student and an intern at Metropolitan Hospital in New York City, if you had a patient who was critically ill and wanted to stay alive it required that you mix and change their IVs during the night shift. For some strange reason, many IVs got plugged up and stopped running after 11 P.M. and were only discovered at about 7 A.M. during morning rounds. We assumed that the night nursing aide staff slowed down all the IVs so that they wouldn't have to keep on changing them or adding life-saving medications to them so that there would be more rest time for the staff.

It was an unwritten rule that if you wanted a very sick patient to make it through the night, you showed up for every four-hour antibiotic IV injection, otherwise you would never be sure if it was given. This total indifference in outlook of city hospital employees in those days was pervasive. It reminds me of some of the horrors that occurred in New Orleans during Hurricane Katrina in 2005, when some of those that stayed behind and didn't evacuate committed crimes of rape, murder, and pillage. Rescue teams were shot at and prevented from doing their jobs. One-third of the police force ran off and some even committed crimes against the very people they had taken an oath to protect.

The indifference in city hospitals also extended to lab workers who routinely wrote "QNS" on specimens (Quantity Not Sufficient) so that they wouldn't have to do tests. To check the honesty of the lab, we would on a weekly basis send water down as a urine specimen. Invariably, it would usually have urine-like values assigned to it on the return lab slip.

One evening we had a trauma victim in the E.R. who needed X-rays immediately. It was 10 P.M. and we stood at the elevator banging and screaming for the operator, who was one floor below. We guessed correctly that we were interrupting his cigarette break. When he finally arrived, rather than help transport the patient, he was ready to do battle with us interns. It was a strange feeling that the lives of the poor people in the ghetto were dependent upon the nurses and nurses' aides that came from the same ghetto. We felt that some of them had a set of ethics far different than ours.

Did we ever catch anyone slowing or turning off an IV? No. Did it occur very frequently? Yes. Were IVs clogged and not functioning in the early morning? Yes. Did the same thing occur in as great a frequency from 7 A.M. to 11 P.M.? No. If it did occur from 7 A.M. to 11 P.M., were we called to fix it during the midnight shift? Rarely.

I haven't worked in a city hospital since 1969 and therefore cannot comment on what's happened since my training. But this much I know: human nature is such that no place can be "assumed" to be a safe haven, least of all hospitals. If you can, choose your hospital carefully. If you can't, fight—and fight hard—or the best, most effective, most expert care you can, wherever you wind up. Bad hospitals are like good garages: the squeaky wheel gets the grease!

The Not-So-Golden Years

THE TEMPLE PORTION of our skull is named from the Latin root, *"tempo"* (translated into English, "time"). That is, it's the first part of man that shows time, in the form of graying. Then the inevitable happens. Hearing starts to go. Shoulders start hunching over and drooping down, and rear ends start sticking outward. Certain ears become highly sensitive to high-pitched noise because of a phenomenon known as "recruitment," which causes a feedback phenomenon in the brain similar to that heard when a microphone echoes and starts to squeal.

Just because these and a host of other less comical, life altering changes take place during the aging process does not mean that our elderly relatives blandly accept them or cherish their independence any less. Now that walking and driving may be much more difficult than ever before, they often refuse to tell their children to take them to their doctor's appointments because they don't want to "bother" them. They admit that they would go out of their way for their children if roles were reversed, and no doubt did so as their children were growing up. No matter, they just don't want to inconvenience the children now that the roles have been reversed and the shoe is on the other foot.

To many old people, independence is everything. They cling to it dearly, sometimes even unwisely, because in many cases it is all that they have left. The last vestige of their independence, if they are drivers, is their cars. And even if they know in their hearts that they are now menaces behind the wheel, they will fight like hell to avoid giving up their licenses. When it was time to keep my mother from driving, we made the mistake of not getting rid of her car. Although she wasn't capable or legally able, she still snuck into the car and took it for a spin around the block on a regular basis.

Eventually for some, the "mental thing" happens. My friend Beverly was moving her mother from Boston to New York to better be able to take care of her during her mother's later years. While they were driving in Bev's car, the mother turned to her and asked who she, Bev, was. How terribly disheartening. The same will happen to many of us, to different degrees, as a parent ages. My mother stopped taking her medicine because she was forgetful and denied that there was anything wrong with her, despite the fact that not taking her medicines kept putting her in the hospital many times.

After a while, their short-term memory goes. It's interesting to observe how their personality takes over when their memory fails. When asked what she had just eaten for breakfast, rather then admitting that she couldn't remember, my mother defiantly replied, "It wasn't good anyway." At that point, driving her any distance was a challenge. First there were the many bathroom stops we had to make for her along the way, even if it was just a few blocks or around the corner. Then there was the recurrent question, "Where are we going?" I bring this up because many children believe that their parents are capable of understanding that they just asked that question. One should never say, "I told you where we are going, a thousand times." That only agitates the parent, who really doesn't remember being told.

Senior Health

HEALTH CHANGES & CONDITIONS RELATED TO AGE

- Heart disease and cerebrovascular diseases will cause 29% of deaths in the elderly.
- Cancer will cause 23% of deaths.
- COPD (chronic obstructive pulmonary disease)[12] and diabetes are the next most prevalent killers on the list.
- Alzheimer's disease—impaired memory, trouble performing familiar tasks, inability to follow directions, loss of basic skills, and eventual dementia—will affect 10% of our senior population and is the seventh leading cause of death in the United States.
- Parkinson's disease, a movement disorder wherein certain brain cells stop carrying or producing dopamine, a chemical produced by the body that helps regulate emotion and physical movement, will affect one out of every three hundred elderly patients.
- Urinary incontinence will affect 38% of women and 17% of men.

---

[12] The umbrella name for a group of chronic lung diseases characterized by irreversible limitation of airflow through the respiratory system, such as emphysema and chronic bronchitis.

- Men develop the "growing" disease, benign prostatic hypertrophy (BPH), a non-cancerous (hence the "benign" in the name) enlargement of the prostate gland that causes weakness of the urinary stream, frequency and urgency of urination, and difficulty in evacuation of urine, eventually leading to urinary tract infection and bladder stones.
- 55% of the elderly (4 times as many women as men) will develop osteoporosis (weak bones caused by a loss of bone density), making them much more susceptible to broken or fractured bones. Risk factors include family history, patients receiving long-term cortisone therapy, (asthmatics, arthritics), and petite or thin Asians or Caucasians. Additionally, drug therapy with heparin (a blood thinner), thyroid medication, aluminum antacids, anticonvulsants, and smoking are pre-disposers to osteoporosis.
- Degenerative arthritis (osteoarthritis) will affect approximately 50% of the elderly.

PRESCRIPTION

- Studies show exercising reduces the pain and subsequent disability of arthritis.
- Studies also show that controlling one's diet (low in cholesterol, saturated and trans fats, and sugar, and high in fiber); diligent management of hypertension, hyperlipidemia, and diabetes; frequent aerobic exercising and cessation of smoking will help prevent, treat, and forestall most of the above-listed causes of diseases and death.
- Weigh yourself daily, or at least every other day.
- Maintain a schedule of annual physicals (and quarterly exams if one has chronic illnesses) for control of blood pressure, cholesterol, and glucose levels.
- Early detection and treatment of Alzheimer's disease can definitely lead to slowing the progress of this terrible disease. Aside from the above listed symptoms, diagnosis is suggested by the "clock test": The patient draws a large clock from memory and is asked to put in the numbers. The patient is then asked to put in the time 2:45 by use of the small and large hands. If the numbers are not put into the correct sequence or are not proportionately

in place, or if the representation of 2:45 is incorrect or irregular, a diagnosis of Alzheimer's follows.

PROGNOSIS

Planning for retirement requires health planning as well as financial planning. The old joke of "if I knew I was going to live this long, I would have taken better care of myself," is no longer a joke. Americans are living longer, with an average life expectancy of 75 years for men and 80 years for women. Health planning includes proper diet, exercise, staying away from bad habits (smoking, drugs), and maintaining good control of blood pressure, cholesterol, and diabetes. To be fully effective, the "plan" must be put into effect at a young age and continued throughout one's life. However, it is never too late to start on the road to a healthier tomorrow.

While aging is referred to as the "golden years," there is a lot to the experience that may tarnish our expectations. As our parents age, they often revert to an inner childhood that makes them outwardly resemble children as well. Make no mistake, this is not an innocent, childlike time for them. It is a grueling, regretful, saddening, maddening experience made doubly so by those of us who don't quite understand what they're going through (but soon will). Patience is the operational word when dealing with all things in life, but particularly when dealing with our elders.

• • •

Miriam Gottlieb, a former patient of mine, was a lovely, slim woman, with short cut, grey hair. She was college educated, a rarity for a woman of 65 back in the early 1970s, and as a result had a great appreciation for opera and the fine arts. She often would trek to the city and later tell me about this and that exhibit she visited or performance she witnessed.

She had never married, and never seemed to regret it. Then along came Harold Schwartz and, after a brief courtship period, they were wed. Within three months, Miriam started complaining. During her bi-monthly visits, I heard complaints of his snoring, his lack of washing, or he did this or he did that. The complaints lasted for three years, stopping abruptly when he died. After a month or two, Miriam started crying at his loss. She would tell me what a great husband he was. When I reminded her of her previously confidential complaining to me, Miriam would deny it emphatically.

Over the next twelve years, as Miriam approached 80, she started to gradually deteriorate. Then, two women in her synagogue's sisterhood organization started taking an interest in her. Both were married and would take turns escorting Miriam to the theatre or an opera performance or a museum. She began to display a new, fresh smile, if just for a short while. I thought it was wonderful that a lonely old woman, living alone, without family, had found people in her life again. When Miriam first told me that she was paying for the tickets and for the transportation for both herself and her escorts, I was shocked and saddened.

I have done work for various charities over the years, and always believed that it didn't matter why a person gave or volunteered. The fact that one contributed was all that counted. Some people gave because they truly believed in the cause, some contributed because they wanted to look important in that social setting. I feel that one gains by helping others—perhaps psychologically, perhaps spiritually. But should they gain monetarily?

Reaching out to a lonely senior can be so rewarding. Perhaps, I thought, the two women just didn't have enough money to purchase their own tickets, and weren't going to let that stop them from doing their "charitable" work. Despite my misgivings, I decided to reserve judgment until all the facts were in.

Unfortunately, Miriam's mental status began to decline. By forgetting to correctly take her medicines, she had frequent bouts of heart failure, requiring multiple hospitalizations. Clearly, Miriam needed to be in a more protective environment; which, for her, meant a nursing home. Miriam had no living relatives, and I felt personally responsible for her well-being. Therefore I obtained her consent. With the permission of her lawyer, I made appointments to visit area nursing homes on my day off.

Immediately I felt just like Goldilocks. The first home was too crowded, the second only interested in how much cash Miriam had. The third was run by an Italian physician. After hearing that a fellow physician was accompanying a patient on his day off, the physician came into the interview personally. He said, quite passionately,

"Please leave Miriam here and I will care for her as you did." We agreed, then went home to make plans.

The next day, Miriam's lawyer called, asking if she was mentally competent.

"Why?" I asked.

Her lawyer quickly explained that Miriam had been convinced by the two women that her money should be "donated" to them, rather then given to the nursing home. After all, they had pointed out, the government would pay the nursing home when her funds ran out.

Taken aback, I phoned the two women to get their side of the story. Each asserted, that "Of course I should take most of Miriam's money." When I pressed them for an explanation, they both explained that they were good "daughters" to Miriam, these past two years, that they "deserved the money."

Did they really!?!

This is a textbook example of elder abuse. When complete strangers start becoming overly friendly with previously ignored elderly neighbors, start spending mysteriously newfound money, or start involving themselves in that person's financial and/or legal affairs, something unsavory is most likely going on. If elder abuse is suspected, call your local, county, or state elder abuse hotline. If physical danger is suspected, call 911.

Don't think that it is only the stranger that preys upon the elderly. As more and more of our parents age, and age poorly, the new wrinkle in a family's comfortable quilt really separates the boys from the men and the girls from the women. I've personally seen children of patients who could certainly win the Terrible Person Prize.

I go out of my way to thank the few families who fully come to the aid of their ill parents. The ones that would drop anything to get their mom or pop to a test or a doctor's appointment, realizing instinctively that, somewhere along the line, the parents had done the same thing for them on many, many occasions. The ones that are always at the bedside, no matter what time of day you make rounds. The ones that make room in their homes for the convalescent phase. These children, who are with their parents 24/7, are few and far between and deserve all the credit society can muster. These are opposed to the ones that drop their sick parent off at the E.R. because they have a "vacation scheduled" and "won't be around to care for them." "We'll be back in a week," they say as they walk out of the E.R. (I should say "skip off," as their footsteps literally lighten and their pace quickens with each step away from those swishing emergency room doors.)

One of the most heart-rending cases I have ever seen involved a woman named Edna. Edna was a lovely, fantastic, dream of a lady. She had just retired from a banking career because she wanted to spend more time with her grandchildren. She read stories on Sunday morning to her church group and volunteered as a "striper" at the local hospital. Then her son lost his job. She offered them the apartment downstairs in her private home. She accepted no rent, of course.

About a month later, the daughter-in-law came in complaining that Edna was "losing it." Edna was "mentally confused" and should "probably be confined to a nursing home," she said. Well, I hadn't noticed any mental change, so I called Edna's minister. "No," he replied, "Edna's doing fine. As a matter of fact, she's actually volunteered to do our books and she's going a great job."

I called the daughter-in-law and told her there must be a mistake, Edna was fine. The next month, a physician called from another town. The daughter-in-law had promptly sought a second opinion. He was quite baffled and wanted to know how well I knew Edna. It was quite clear what was going on. Another month went by and Edna came into the office for her quarterly evaluation and she happily said that her son convinced her to sign her house over to him. Now it was she who was living in the downstairs apartment, in her own home, and not the other way around. To help her son out, she was also now paying rent, where before she had refused to take the same from her son.

Had Edna, in fact, lost it? Far from it. She knew *exactly* what was going on; she just wanted to be with her grandchildren. About a year later, the son sold the house and he and his family moved to South Carolina. Edna stayed behind and took an apartment because she still had her church and friends up here. I hadn't seen Edna for three months or so, when one day I got a phone call from a nursing home in South Carolina asking if I would mind sending any pertinent records on their new patient. As you might have guessed, their new patient was dear old Edna.

• • •

I am sad to say that there are many, many cases like this one and like Miriam's. In this society, we have to a great degree lost our connection to our elders. We hide them away in old folks' homes, force them into retirement, and generally try to forget they exist. But exist they do. And they are a vital source of wisdom and a powerful opportunity for service. And let's not forget we will be elders ourselves one day. If we watch out for our elders, and treat them with the respect they deserve, we will not only be more able to protect them—we just might change the way we deal with elders in time for our golden years, when we'll need it most!

Elder Abuse

DIAGNOSIS

According to the U.S. Administration on Aging: "The older population—persons 65 years or older, numbered 36.3 million in 2004 (the latest year for which data is available). They represented 12.4% of the U.S. population, about one in every eight Americans. By 2030 there will be about 71.5 million older persons, more than twice their number in 2000. People 65+ represented 12.4% of the population in the year 2000 but are expected to grow to be 20% of the population by 2030."

Clearly, old age will be an issue for all of us in the future, but only if we're lucky. We need to be vigilant of—and for—our elders, whether related to us or not. It helps to keep in mind that old age is a privilege we earn; the number of tragic deaths in younger years makes it clear how lucky we are to even reach old age. And despite the fact that the progression of age brings with it certain inevitable declines in physical functions, it in no way means that an older person lacks in other areas, such as social merit or even basic humanity. Our elders should be honored, not ignored; revered, not wasted.

• • •

SIGNS AND SYMPTOMS OF ELDER ABUSE
• Financial abuse:
  1. Overly friendly strangers begin to appear in the lives of older people; or neighbors, friends, and family members suddenly start spending newfound money or explicitly lay claims to the elder's money.

2. People start to insist on having their name included on all accounts.
3. Checks are being cashed without permission of the elder.
4. Personal belongings begin to disappear.
5. Doctor's appointments are not being kept.
6. Unusual items charged on a credit card.
7. Power of attorney suddenly becomes an issue for no visible reason.
- Emotional/physical abuse:
  1. There is a gradual change in the individual from calm to emotional upset, and sometimes even an appearance of emotional disturbance.
  2. Their behavior becomes more nervous, more demanding.
  3. They become negative, agitated, and increasingly angry.
- Signs/characteristics of a potential elder abuser:
  1. An abuser can be someone "talking down" to the abused or calling them names.
  2. The abuser makes attempts to withdraw the abused from family and friends.[13]

PRESCRIPTION

- Detection of elder abuse, be it financial, psychological, sexual, or nursing home–specific, may depend upon you.
- If elder abuse is suspected, call your local, regional, or state Elder Abuse Hotline.
- If physical danger is suspected, call 911.
- The National Center for Elder Abuse and the National Committee for Prevention of Elderly Abuse sponsor many programs.
- Domestic violence programs in every community offer shelter as well as crisis lines and support groups; mental health and counseling services and associations are available to determine

---

[13] I observed one such case which involved my children's former nanny. When she passed away at the age of 80 her husband's family, who hadn't been heard from in over twenty years, abducted him from his home. He was brought, weak and aged, to a nursing home in North Carolina. When they learned one month later that he had no money and wasn't going to get his wife's estate, he was quickly brought back to his New York apartment. They were never heard from again.

whether the elder is capable of meeting their own needs and to discuss available options and resources.

- The Older American's Act established a network of free legal services for persons over the age of 60.
- You do not need absolute proof to report suspected abuse, nor do you have to give your name; all calls are handled confidentially.
- When all else fails, call the Eldercare Locator service of the U.S. Administration on Aging: 1-800-677-1116.

PROGNOSIS

In this society we have, to a great degree, lost our connection to our elders. We hide them away in old folks' homes, force them into retirement, and generally try to forget they exist. But exist they do, and they are a vital source of wisdom and a powerful opportunity for service. And let's not forget we will be elders ourselves one day.

There are two million reported cases of elder abuse in the United States each year, and it is estimated that eight million more cases go unreported. As good neighbors, if we take the time to check on our seniors we will be paying them back for their lifetime efforts. Community, counseling, and educational resources are available for those who are mentally capable. For the others, all they have is us.

If we watch out for our elders and treat them with the respect they deserve, we will not only be better able to protect them—we just might change the way we deal with elders in time for our golden years, when we'll need it most.

A Sensible Hope

WHEN A PATIENT OF MINE WENT TO AN ONCOLOGIST, he or she would be bombarded with statistics that would practically knock your socks off. "You have a ninety-eight percent chance of dying if you don't take the chemo" and "a ten percent chance of living if you do." And, as if that weren't enough "good news," they would shortly thereafter hear the following caveat: "Your hair is going to fall out, you'll be sick most of the time, and there's a good chance you won't make it." Patients ran back to me horrified. The message conveyed was clear: they were dying and were told there was no chance of survival. They were hysterical. Clearly, cancer is an onerous subject with damnable odds. But what my patients were responding to was not so much the disease as the delivery.

Just as there are things I would like you to know about certain illnesses and life stages so you can more effectively deal with and overcome them, there are things we all need to know about death, the one medical scenario we will all face and which is just as much a part of life as anything else.

A lot of things have changed between when I first entered practice and today, some thirty-six (gulp!) years later. In the old days, if a patient was dying there were always family members who would say, "Don't tell them, they wouldn't be able to take the news. It would kill them." It was strange, but like the Army there was this duplicitous "don't ask, don't tell" atmosphere. I know that if I were in and out of the hospital for months, losing weight, getting all sorts of injections, I'd want to know quite simply what was going on. But in those days patients didn't ask; instead they silently accepted your efforts. Deep down, I assumed they understood but were overwhelmed by the fear and finality of hearing the truth out loud. Rarely, when someone did ask about their illness, they seemed to block whatever you told them anyway, as if you never said it to begin with.

The physician having to dance around or avoid the truth with someone who was dying? It wasn't a healthy relationship in any way. Not for the doctor, not for the nurse, not for the family, certainly not for the patient.

There was usually an unspoken pact with the family. If they said, "don't let them suffer" or that it was time to "pull the plug," the decision was done altogether, no questions asked. If there was no hope for Mrs. Jones, it was discussed with all the options with the family and *not* the complacent patient. The IVs would be slowed down, the respirator stopped, and the patient allowed to die naturally without heroic long-term interference. I could never, ever think of giving someone something to end his or her life. But I could withhold therapy in good conscience if I thought there was no chance of survival or, barring that, recovery of some kind of life quality.

Alternatively, many a hospitalized patient would say, "I want to die" or "I don't want to go on anymore." Kiddingly, with sort of a straight face, I would always retort, "For $5, I can make it happen." Whether they questioned my sanity or knew I was trying to lighten their feelings, not one out of a thousand or so patients ever offered the $5. The point is, practically no one really *wants* to die. In fact, it's human instinct to want to live, for as long as possible. But death, like life, is a harsh taskmaster, and we must be prepared for the inevitable. And it is just one of our doctor's many jobs to help us do just that.

Just as with any profession, in medicine there are certain types of personalities that choose their various sub-specialties. Every neurologist I have ever met has the same bland, non-responsive affect. Talking to them is like talking to a wall; you feel your words just bouncing off of them and falling on the floor. Oncologists, whose life's work it is to deal with people suffering from a disease that causes thirteen percent of deaths worldwide and which will affect approximately one out of every three of us, are usually unemotional personalities as well; a good survival mechanism for the field they ultimately chose. Many of their patients have horrible diseases and will die, so reading off a litany of statistics about life or death is part of their daily routine and, as a result, is done matter-of-factly.

Often a patient will run back to my office hyper-anxious and upset, saying the oncologist told them they were "going to die." After calming the patients down, I usually say something to the effect that many people will die, but the doctor did say that they have a chance of making it, that the cancer was caught early enough or had not spread enough. This gives them time to fully grasp what's going on and allows them a chance to calmly intellectualize the process. Then they will be psychologically prepared and better able to make rational decisions.

Once, an English gentleman showed up at my door—a transplanted IBM scientific type—asking if his wife, in the hospital for two weeks with ovarian cancer, was going to live or die. I was sort of taken back by the abrupt directness of his response. I answered, "I don't think she'll live much longer."

He said, "Very well, I just wanted to know" and left before I could sit him down and comfort him. He was a rarity and he could do well with the number-crunching, fact-giving, types of physicians. But most people need compassion and warmth.

Ideally, there should be some wiggle room for the physician to artfully help his patients navigate this new, uncharted avenue of their lives. Unfortunately, we are in the era of litigation and signed informed medical consents. Nowadays, if a patient is on the verge of dying; we need DNR (do not resuscitate) forms, signed proof of a living will, *and* a medical proxy. We aren't allowed to "pull the plug" with their own and their family's consent, and the "final treatment" becomes less of a medical decision and more like a legal fiat. I won't even dignify with discussion the ultra-conservative movement's drive to deny people the right to die with dignity by forcing life sustaining measures upon them.

The fact is we are all going to go through this experience called death. The more we learn to embrace it, the more healing and enriching this experience will be. In some primitive tribes, death is viewed as a sacred ritual, something that the whole village participates in— including the children. It is not something outside of life, but an integral part of it. When you think about it, death is the most certain thing about life. And it is also one of the most powerful experiences. If we can learn to honor, respect, and even celebrate the transition from this world to the next, we will not only fear death much less ... we will start living life much more.

FINAL OFFICE ROUNDS

IN THE PREVIOUS PAGES, I'VE TRIED TO SHARE some of the most meaning-ful knowledge I've gleaned from thirty-five years of medical prac-tice. Key among these insights is that patients are human beings with thoughts, feelings, hopes, and fears. They are obviously vulnerable when they come to a doctor with potential symptoms of a life-threat-ening illness such as cancer or heart disease. But there is more often simply a sense of helplessness at the realization that they are not in control of their circumstances, that they must rely on someone else to cure them. And this experience cuts across age, race, economic, and social status. They could be a mover and shaker of our society; a mega-successful businessman, a movie star, a politician, whatever. But in their doctor's office or in the hospital, they are just Mr. or Mrs. Whomever in room 719.

It is at once humbling and extremely frightening.

Another key insight, one I want you to take away above all else, is that doctors are human too. I say this not to let my fellow colleagues off the hook, but to protect you, the patient, from the mistakes that can be made when you believe your doctor is infallible—or, worse, when your doctor believes he is! The fact is that doctors come to this partnership carrying their own baggage (sometimes an entire mono-grammed set of Samsonite). And it is ultimately up to you, the patient, to determine if they're qualified and competent to help you. Are they knowledgeable or caring enough? Will they stay on top of your case? Do they create a safe environment where you feel com-fortable sharing your deepest thoughts and concerns? Will they pro-tect you, as the captain of the medical ship, from the often rough seas of the hospital environment?

In this complex mix of patients' needs and fears, as well as those of physicians, there has to be a way for both to unite positively. And that, finally, is the true aim of this book: to begin a dialogue that will help you and your doctor create a powerful partnership for achieving optimal health. Your physician must be able to hear you, understand you, and use all of your cues to come up with a fitting and effective diagnosis and a treatment plan. But you, the patient, are not along for a free ride. As it is the physician's role to cure, it is the modern patient's role to be an active participant. You are empowered to protect yourself and always be on the alert for mistakes. But you must be on a quest to know all there is to know about your illness and your options. You are not a passenger, but the co-pilot, along with your doctor, on this flight toward total well-being. It's not always a smooth ride. There will likely be some choppy weather and turbulence, and you may even get off the flight plan at times.

But a long as you and your doctor continue to navigate together, you will make the necessary course corrections to keep you on track toward your destination and hopefully and happily guide you to that safe landing of true and lasting health.

ABOUT THE AUTHOR

RICHARD S. KLEIN, M.D., is a practicing physician in Yorktown Heights, New York, specializing in internal medicine and infectious diseases. He also holds the position of Associate Professor of Medicine at the New York Medical College and serves on the board of the Westchester County (NY) Department of Health.

His career began as a corpsman in the military, where he received several commendations for his work as a Marine Corps field medic. He was inspired to attend medical school by his experience in the military, and went on to study medicine at the University of Rome, one of the oldest universities in the Western world.

In the years since, Dr. Klein has run for Congress in New York's 19th Congressional District, receiving an endorsement from the *New York Times* for his "immense sense of service and volunteerism to the community at large." He is presently involved with a multitude of volunteer organizations serving the community. He has been the fire surgeon for the Yorktown Heights Fire Department for the last two decades and is board member and physician for My Sisters Place and the Northern Westchester Shelter, both of which serve battered women and children. Dr. Klein also donates an annual scholarship to the *Circolo DaVinci*, an organization that promotes Italian heritage, as a way of paying back the worldwide Italian community for affording him the opportunity to study medicine in Italy. As an instrument rated aircraft pilot, Dr. Klein has volunteered for Angel Flight, an organization that flies cancer patients and their families, free of charge, to distant treating hospitals.

Dr. Klein has been knighted by the Italian government and received medals and awards from the Israeli and Egyptian governments in recognition of his efforts on behalf of each of those countries' citizens. In addition to this volume, he is the author of *The Wine Tasters Album* and founder of the Doctor's Fast diet system. A father of two adult daughters, Dr. Klein currently lives with his wife, Caryn; his ten-year-old daughter, Arianna; and his one and a half-year-old son, Matthew, in Somers, New York.